YOUR WEIGHT OR YOUR LIFE?

Your Weight

or

Your Life?

Balancing the Scale for a Healthy Life from Within

BARBARA MCCALMON

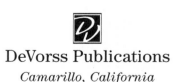

DeVorss Publications
Camarillo, California

09/09

Library of Congress Control Number: 2006921862

ISBN10: 0875168213
ISBN13: 9780875168210

First DeVorss Edition, 2006

Printed in the United States of America

DeVorss & Company, Publisher
P.O. Box 1389
Camarillo, California 93011-1389
www.devorss.com

*To my husband Kevin
for his voice of reason and
support when I found myself
out on a limb.*

*To my mother
for her commitment,
wisdom, and strength.*

*To my sister Marilyn
for her ever-present generosity of
spirit and encouragement.*

CONTENTS

PREFACE

It was the day after Easter, and I was rifling through the refrigerator for a piece of fruit to take to work. As I closed the door, I noticed all the food left over from the previous day. There was the usual ham and scalloped potatoes, but all the tempting items—chocolate Easter bunnies, jelly beans, and cake—were still sitting on the counter.

Many years earlier I would never have been able to view those sweets with such indifference. They would have been quickly consumed in one of my frequent eating binges. Now, as I viewed them with such detachment, I felt an overwhelming sense of gratitude, even awe, that I was at last rid of the compulsion. Finally, I was not fearful of being powerless around easily accessible food. For some reason on this particular day I experienced an epiphany. I knew with deep conviction that food would never again have a stranglehold on my life, but would instead assume its proper role as simply a pleasurable experience.

I could not have felt that way thirteen years earlier, even after I was released from the Rader Institute for Eating Disorders, and certainly not in the years prior to entering the Institute when my life was so severely crippled by my eating obsession.

For most people, eating is enjoyable. The family dinner table is usually a place of conviviality and fellowship, where food usually brings out the best in everyone. That is its proper role in our lives. But when food becomes an obsession, as it had in my case, conviviality, friendship and humor have no part in the eating experience. There is only misery.

I am writing this book with the hope of demonstrating that no matter how desperate a problem may appear, there is always a solution to that problem. One need only develop faith in their Higher Power—and in themselves—to bring balance back into their lives. It is then that peace and joy will finally return to them.

BARBARA MCCALMON
Broomfield, Colorado

ACKNOWLEDGMENTS

I wish to acknowledge my deepest appreciation to the Mile Hi Church of Religious Science, which has been an inspiration and a beacon of light to me when I needed its teachings most, as well as to *Science of Mind* magazine for its Daily Guides that have also helped guide and enrich my life. I am also grateful to the Rader Institute for Eating Disorders for placing me on the road to recovery from a terrible addiction. I wish to offer special thanks to Cliff Johnson, of Cliff Johnson & Associates, who undertook the editing of this book with enthusiasm and made many helpful contributions.

Last, but certainly not least, I want to extend my debt of gratitude to my sister Marilyn, to Dr. Hans Kuisle, who was instrumental in advancing our medically-based spas, and to the men and women who pass through our doors. It is their willingness to care for themselves through massage, proper skin care, and nutrition that keeps me inspired. Special thanks also go to my own clients and staff who have been so loyal and steadfast during our growth over the years.

CHAPTER 1

My Early Years

I have always considered myself a normal, happy child during my early years. Now that I view this period as an adult, I see how dysfunctional my childhood really was, and how it led to my overwhelming obsession with food. During these years, my father was an active alcoholic, and due to his drinking our family environment was not exactly healthy. Of course, it was largely because of his drinking that there was seldom enough money for us to live decently. True, we generally had basic food items in the house, but "luxury" food such as snacks were absent—and, at times, we had simply no food at all. As children we resorted to gathering pop bottles around the neighborhood to sell at the grocery store in an effort to eat.

One Saturday afternoon our grandparents surprised us with a visit. They were retired farmers who lived in the small town of Brush, Colorado, some ninety miles away. They were not wealthy by any means and survived on a small Social Security pension. At the time, Dad was in the local bar. My grandfather happened to open the refrigerator and was shocked to discover only two eggs and a little milk. Mom was planning to make pancakes for dinner because there was simply nothing else in the house. Again, we had no money for food. Despite his own limited income, grandpa gave my mother twenty dollars. I do not remember what we finally ate for dinner, but I do recall that my mother was terribly grateful for the money, which enabled us to buy food for several days. Twenty dollars went a long way in those days.

Since I had been deprived of food for so many years, it became an obsession for me. If I was fortunate enough to find it in plentiful supply, I would simply eat and continue to eat. At the time I was an active child; quite lean, and usually hungry. I had many friends in the neighborhood who always seemed to have an abundance of groceries in their houses, so when food was offered, I indulged myself, usually until it was gone. A bag of corn chips or a box of doughnuts did not last long within my reach.

One Sunday afternoon, when I was about eight years old, my mother took us to a gathering at the home of a family friend. I immediately spied a huge spread of food. In no time at all I was going back for second and third portions. When I was returning with my fourth plate of food, my brother mentioned that I needed to quit because I was beginning to act and look like a little glutton. I did stop— but only because of my brother's comment—not because I did not want more food. Although I should have been full, what eight-year old child can eat four plates of food and still be hungry?

A few years after this unhappy occurrence, our family was invited to an event in connection with my father's work. All I remember of the occasion was the massive number of glazed doughnuts. I am certain I must have eaten at least fifteen of them. Although at the time I did not recognize it, I know now that my overindulgence was a futile attempt to fill a void in me that was far more psychological than physical. It was a need that only in my later years I recognized and would seriously address.

Since I was an active child and was unable to overeat at home (simply because there was not enough food), my weight never became a problem until many years later. I remember being hungry often. I would visit the neighbors, an older couple, and ask them for food. I remember seeing the woman of the house sitting on the couch, smoking long, filtered cigarettes and continually coughing. I learned a few years later that she died of emphysema. Bill was her white-haired husband whom I got to know best. Though he was sometimes uncomfortable with children, he seemed to like me. Knowing that I was hungry much of the time, he would let me go down to their basement where they stored their food, to find something to eat. Bill was employed at the nearby Army base. He purchased groceries from the commissary. All I remember is that he had bags and bags full of food (quite tempting to the imagination of a six-year-old), mostly canned goods and crackers. I soon developed a particular fondness for Ritz crackers. After I would have my fill of crackers, I would return home or wait until my friends were available to play.

Several times a week I wound up over at Bill's house scrounging for something more than Ritz crackers. I always regretted that he never had any peanut butter. (Of course, we never had peanut butter at our house!) So, I would leave with a stomach full of Ritz crackers. Needless to say I will not eat a Ritz cracker to this day.

During this time I do not have a memory of Mom being around much. She worked a hard double shift waitressing at the airport to help keep food on the table and a roof over our heads. Although my alcoholic father did work, he spent most of his earnings in the bars after work, before work, and sometimes during work.

My sister Marilyn was five years my senior. Though she had friends from junior high school, she always seemed busy with them and seldom brought them home. When Dad was home, he was usually drunk and, as a result, Mom was angry and unpleasant. Not exactly a situation Marilyn wanted her friends to see!

My brother Mike, two years older than me, was artistic, smart and a good athlete. He was truly gifted. When my father was sober, he had nothing but praise for him. However, when Dad was drinking, it was quite another story. If Mike stepped out of line, he treated him cruelly. Once Mike and his friends broke into an empty house in the neighborhood. When Dad got wind of it, he beat the holy hell out of my brother. It still bothers me to this day.

I truly admired and respected my brother and his talent and did everything I could to get him to like me, but he never returned my affection. If he talked to me at all, it was in a critical way. One Sunday morning, my mother had gone to church. My sister Marilyn was in charge, I must have been about seven. Mike and I had the comics spread out on the living room floor. Mike was insisting that I fold them up perfectly. When I failed to do this to his satisfaction, he grew so enraged that he loaded his BB gun with an ink cartridge and shot me in the knee with it. Blood and ink spurted out of my knee. I was crying hysterically just about the time Mom walked in the door. She grabbed the gun and broke it over her knee on the spot. There was so much anger and pain in our home at that time.

Marilyn was my biggest supporter. I was naturally athletic, and when I won a blue ribbon for broad jump in the first grade, I remember how proud she was of me. I wanted to be on the cheerleading squad in the third grade, but I had to have a uniform. Unfortunately, we could not afford the cost of one. My mom did the best she could, though she searched in vain in used clothing stores to find the dark blue leggings and sweater that were required. Though I was embarrassed when I showed up to practice, because I didn't look like the rest of the girls, I never connected this deprivation to my father or blamed him for our problems.

CHAPTER 2

GROWING UP AND
GROWING HEAVIER

For me the sun rose and set on my father. He was my idol. In spite of his drinking, he spoiled me as much as he could. I was his blonde-haired, blue-eyed little girl. He took me many places with him, including the bars. I loved it. At the time, I didn't know he had a problem; I just loved being with him. He didn't take my older brother and sister. I think they were aware of his problem and did not want to be around him when he was drinking. Not me! I lived to be with my daddy. I remember being with him many early Saturday mornings in those dingy bars. While he would be drinking, the waitresses would keep me busy with huge plates of pancakes and syrup. What could be better? I was with my father and was able to fill my hungry stomach.

Sometimes, later in the day, he would take me to McDonald's. McDonald's was my favorite place. I loved seeing those golden arches come into view through the windshield. I would get so excited at the thought of eating a hamburger, fries, and chocolate shake. I loved dipping my hot fries into that cold shake and savoring the flavor.

I was starting to really love food. I was still a very lean little girl and very active. My sister and friends and I would sometimes spend all day at the neighborhood pool in the summer. Every once in a while my sister or I would make a dollar from selling pop bottles or Dad would give us money. When he had money, he could be generous. Candy bars were then only a dime, so we would buy ten Butterfinger or Baby Ruth bars at the snack bar at the pool and eat them all between us throughout the afternoon.

One late afternoon, while my father and I were driving home from his day of drinking, he put me on his lap and asked me to steer the car and keep it on the wide road while he worked the pedals. Obviously he was too drunk to be able to drive the car straight, so he relied on me. I did well. We made it home safe and sound, and I was excited to tell my mom the news of my first driving experience. As soon as I shared my story, I sensed some tension between my mother and father. I was disappointed that she was not as excited about my driving as I was! Soon after that, my outings with my father came to an end. I didn't understand it until I was much older. I just remember being mad at my mother for depriving me of the pleasure of going out with my father.

Not too long after this event my parents separated. I recall that one day my father was just gone. Mom told me he had to go away because he was sick and needed some time to get better. I was devastated. I remember going down into the spare bedroom in the basement, which I was deathly afraid of any other time, and crying for what seemed like hours. I wanted to be alone in my pain. I particularly did not want to be teased by my older brother and sister and made to feel embarrassed because of my sadness over my father's disappearance.

Eventually, my father returned home, and a few months later my mom was pregnant with my little brother, Timothy. My mother also joined Al-Anon in an effort to cope with my father's drinking.

I had a friend named Debbie. They lived a block from us, and I loved going over to her house because they always had potato chips, Coke and plenty of snacks. One beautiful sunny afternoon Debbie and I went over to her house and opened large bag of corn chips. We ate the entire bag, and I managed more than two-thirds of it. I was so sick afterwards that I never touched another corn chip until I was in high school.

I noticed that Debbie had severe scars from burns on her hands, arms and back. When I asked her about them, she told me her mother had accidentally bathed her in water that was too hot. Her father was often angry and yelling at her mother. One afternoon, when Debbie and I came inside the house from playing, we walked into a war zone. Her father was screaming at her mother and her mother was screaming back at him. Then he suddenly pushed her mother into the kitchen wall causing the toaster to fall to the floor, and sparks flew from the still lighted appliance. At once her mom picked up the toaster and threw it at her father, barely missing Debbie and me. I was very scared. Her father screamed at me to go home; this I did, gladly.

I had never witnessed such violence before, and it remained in my memory for a long time. My father was home when I walked in from Debbie's house, and I told my parents what I had witnessed. He said I was not allowed to go to Debbie's house anymore; if I wanted to play with her, she would have to come to our house. Of course, I knew that this also meant no more snacks! Later, Debbie and her brothers were removed from their home by a social service worker. They would be returned a few weeks later, only to be taken away again and again. I still wonder about the future of that family. I sense it was not a happy one. All their children were abused, and Debbie had the scars to prove it.

We moved to Texas during the summer between my third and fourth grade in school. Happily, my father quit drinking during that year we were in Texas. My younger brother, Timothy, was not quite a year old. You would think that at my young age of eight, I would have had fun with this new, tiny member of the household. I didn't. I resented him terribly. Not only was I no longer the youngest, I had to hang his wet diapers on the clothesline after Mom washed them. I am ashamed to admit that I actually attempted to drown him once. I thank God that my attempt failed. We were playing in the kiddy pool in our back yard, and he kept playfully putting his face in the water and blowing into it. It looked so tempting to hold his little head under the water for a while. Though I did force his head under for few seconds, I suddenly realized what I was doing and stopped. Today, I am glad that I stopped when I did. I now deeply love my younger brother, and I would not now have my perfect niece and nephew if I had carried through on my hateful act.

By this time, money was more abundant, and so were snack foods around our house. I was also lonely and bored because my old friends were gone and I had not met any new ones. Food became my companion. My weight began to increase, and I started fourth grade as the chubby little girl from Colorado.

And so it went. We moved to Chicago in the summer of the following year. I also began to put on more weight. Unfortunately, my father started drinking again. And I found I was not his blonde-haired, blue-eyed, lean little girl anymore. My hair had darkened, and I started fifth grade weighing 164 pounds. A lot of weight for someone standing only five feet, one inch tall! The good news was I still made friends and had fun in school. Most of my friends were in the "In Crowd." Two of them were to become cheerleaders, and I felt accepted by them. Boys liked me well enough. A few of my classmates made fun of me, but it was not unbearable. I can only assume I had a likable enough personality to make me reasonably popular. However, the one person who continued to tease me was my older brother, Mike. "Log legs" was his favorite expression. I did want to be thin, and I envied the girls who had such cute little figures.

At the end of my seventh grade year, my mom convinced me to join Weight Watchers. Despite the fact that Dad had started to sober up again and money was tight, my mother was a saint and very supportive. She worked overtime in the kitchen preparing the meals I needed to eat with the family. However, by the time school started I had lost twenty-five pounds. I still had fifteen or more pounds to go, but I certainly looked and felt better about myself. Every morning before school I would prepare my lunch for the day, a tuna fish and mustard sandwich with a piece of fruit. Tuna fish was not packed in water then, so I ate this oily tuna and mustard concoction on white bread. I enviously watched while all my friends ate their hot lunches of lasagna or hamburger and fries, followed by an ice cream bar. Nevertheless, I was not to be swayed. I stayed on my diet, only occasionally indulging in french fries or cookies.

One day while cleaning out my closet I found two bags of butterscotch candy. I was surprised at how little I cared about eating them and more surprised that I had lost the desire for them. The fact that I was having a lot of fun in school, and getting some positive attention from the male species, really helped keep my mind off of food and the promise of its instant gratification. With my sister's and mother's encouragement, I joined an all-women's exercise studio. I was dedicated. Three times a week after school, I would walk to the studio and do my routine of sit-ups, leg lifts, and whatever else they prescribed. Then I would walk the two miles home. That exercise really boosted my ability to lose weight and tone up. I was starting to wear more stylish clothes and feel really good about being a female.

One day, walking home from the exercise studio, I learned about the not-so-positive attention from men. It was a nice sunny afternoon and I was about a mile from my home. I was wearing a cute little outfit and was feeling good about myself. I noticed a young man walking toward me on the same side of the street. As we passed each other, we both smiled. Then the next thing I knew he was running up behind me, and suddenly grabbed me. However, I acted on pure adrenaline, pushed him away from me as hard as I could and started to run. He ran after me, but I was able to distance myself from him because he was wearing high-heeled boots that slowed him. The chase lasted for nearly half a mile before he finally gave up. In any case, it was a frightening experience.

We moved again at the end of my eighth-grade year. I managed to stay busy helping my mother get our new house cleaned and painted. My father had finally quit drinking for good this time, and we left my older sister Marilyn and brother Mike in Chicago to pursue their own interests. My older brother Michael had agreed to rejoin us before school started.

I had not made any new friends yet that summer. I was so busy helping my mother that I did not have time to make food my companion. I started ninth grade actually thinner than I had ever been—perhaps a size 12. I joined the track team and became involved in some minor competitions. I also met my friend Lynn that year. We remained good friends all through high school. We met a lot of boys, enjoyed some fun times, and managed to involve ourselves in some of the troubles of normal school girls.

When I became a junior I was eligible for a vocational program in cosmetology training as long as I maintained a 3.0 average and put in the required training hours. I had my cosmetology license by the time I graduated. I loved the idea of having an occupation upon graduation to support myself, because I knew I would never go to collage. It was simply not in the family budget. During the last two years of high school, I went to cosmetology school in the mornings, high school classes in the afternoons, and I worked about twenty-five hours a week at a local restaurant. I stayed very busy. My sister had moved back home in my junior year and found an apartment not far from our home.

As many girls do in cosmetology school, I colored my hair. I went from to true brunette to a bleached blonde. My sister decided that since it looked so good on me, maybe we could bleach her hair as well. So I gathered together all the necessary supplies for the "operation." However, after three hours into the process, it was turning into a disaster. When I left her apartment that night, Marilyn had orange-pink hair! I spent the next night coloring it back to the natural color. We still laugh about her orange hair to this day.

I also found time to spend time with Lynn and go boy hunting at the local hangout for all the schools in the area. During this time my weight seemed to go down; at times I even managed to fit into a size ten. It was not something I set out to do, it was just that my life was so busy and fun during these years. I found I did not have time to eat—or should I say, overeat. Although I would occasionally binge, such splurges did not seem to really affect me much. The binges were so rare and unexpected, I found myself ignoring them. I also found that after a binge, I wasn't hungry for several days so I would simply not eat. It all seemed so easy! I was shortly to discover how wrong I was.

CHAPTER 3

MARRIAGE

That discovery came one night at a hamburger restaurant where I was working. It started with an eating binge that really scared me, because I did not think anyone would be capable of eating the amount of food I did that night. After the restaurant closed, three of us were responsible for making sure the grill and floors were clean and everything was ready for the opening crew in the morning. As was true many nights, there was always a large number of hamburgers, cheeseburgers, and fish sandwiches left over from the last minute evening rush. On this particular night, there were some twenty unsold hamburgers and a few fish sandwiches.

We were allowed to eat the leftover inventory, just so long as it was recorded in our waste record. Well, to this day I do not know what obsession came over me. I ate a cheeseburger while I was cleaning, followed by another, then another, and another. When the cleanup was completed, I discovered I had eaten twelve cheeseburgers and two fish sandwiches! I was the one responsible for telling the manager how much inventory was left over. However, I was so ashamed that I lied and told him that only eight hamburgers and one fish sandwich were consumed. I knew that if he happened to look in the inventory bucket he would learn of my unhealthy appetite. This was something I did not want anyone to know.

That binge bothered me for many days to follow. And I made sure never to let it happen again—well, for a while, anyway. I also remember many episodes during my high school years of not eating at all for three or four days. What I was doing, of course, was preparing myself for another eating binge.

In time I graduated from high school and, a month later, passed my cosmetology license. I could now embark on a career of manicuring, pedicuring, and acrylic fingernail application. However, six months after landing my first job, my father died of cancer. I had just turned nineteen. I am not sure whether it was because of my youth or my embarking on a new career, but I really never gave myself time to grieve his death. Also, at this time I met a young man whom I would eventually marry. We really had little in common except that we both had alcoholic fathers. Unlike his father, mine became sober and turned into a wonderful father and husband when I was eleven. He was never abusive or mean to me in any way. Though, as his drinking progressed, he could become indifferent and sarcastic. However, because of my youth, it seemed to make little impact on me. As far as I was concerned, he was the father I loved with all my heart.

As I mentioned earlier, my mother had joined Al-Anon and was active in the program for several years. The Al-Anon program really helped my mother retain her sanity. She seemed much happier and serene even after my father started drinking again in Chicago. Then, by some miracle my father took his last drink on Thanksgiving Day, a month before my twelfth birthday. He embarked on the Alcoholics Anonymous twelve-step program and our family truly began the process of healing and became somewhat functional by the time he died.

During my father's years of sobriety, my parents' marriage blossomed. I am now so grateful I was gifted with the opportunity to witness a healthy, successful marriage between them. We had many wonderful family evenings, and their sense of humor had a way of filtering down to the rest of us.

My own life at the time was not so lucky. I chose to marry Rick, a man whose father was an active drinker and mother a true victim and co-dependent. Unknowingly, I had laid in my husband's lap my sense of well-being and happiness and made it his responsibility to maintain it. That is quite a tall order for a fellow who came from a dysfunctional family himself. Is it any wonder that he could not make me happy?

Rick was also a liar. At times he would lie even when it was easier to tell the truth. I once happened to overhear a conversation he was having with his mother. He told her he had a bowl of soup for lunch, when I knew for a fact that he had eaten a sandwich. That baffled me, so I started to pay closer attention to his statements and caught him in many more lies.

He was also jealous and accusatory. Rick questioned everything I did. If I came home twenty minutes later than expected, he was convinced I was cheating on him. Perhaps it was his own his guilt over past indiscretions. Soon I discovered that he had been carrying on a long-distance relationship with his ex-girlfriend. It was then I decided to leave him, but not without some drama. Once he realized I was leaving, he hid the keys to my car and even the distributor cap to his own car in case I tried to leave while he was out drinking with his buddies.

However, I was one step ahead of him. Unbeknownst to him, I had an extra set of keys to my car, quickly loaded it with some essential items and went to my mother's. However, he had made one fatal error. He hid the distributor cap from his own car in mine, which was now thirty minutes away at my mother's house! He failed to see the humor in this. He arrived at my mother's house the next day, threatening to burn it down if I did not come back.

Did that tactic work? Decidedly not! However, I had gained forty-five pounds in the brief year we were married. Food, once again, had become my lover and companion. Is it any wonder I was living a total lie on every level in my marriage? How can you know or love someone when you cannot trust what they say? I found it impossible.

Also, I found that I was incapable of truly liking myself during my brief marriage to Rick. I also discovered myself lying to him because of his controlling and suspicious nature. Once again, my love for food came to my rescue. All I wanted to do was eat. That was the only thing that gave me pleasure.

I found myself complaining about everything. Looking back on those days, I now see how incredibly negative I was. In reality, I was simply lazy about making my life better, though I certainly did not like it the way it was. Of course, I knew I had to get out of my marriage, and when I told Rick I was leaving, he broke down and cried. It was the first time I really felt close to him. He was truly in pain and was not afraid to expose his hurt. Though it was the only time I felt we had honestly shared something, it was too little and too late. I was unable to live with someone I could not trust.

During this time I had been working at a little salon across from our apartment building. I was busy there, and it seemed I was the only one who really had any clients. When I left Rick, I temporarily moved home with my mother. I was grateful to have this job. One Monday morning, I arrived at work at nine sharp, opened up the front door to the salon and found it totally empty! It was an incredible shock, to say the least! I later discovered the owner had run into severe financial difficulties and was forced to close down. However, she had been good enough to leave the phone sitting on the floor, and I immediately called my mother in a panic. I did not know what to do. I had booked ten clients that day and found myself with no equipment. It would only be a matter of minutes before they would start coming through the door.

By some miracle I found the owner's phone number and called her. She asked me to come to her home a few minutes away, where she supplied me with enough product to get me started—as well as my appointment book. I piled everything in my car and began to drive around looking for a place to work in the area. I soon found another small salon a few miles away, walked in and told the receptionist my story of woe. A pretty blond woman overheard my conversation and poked her head out of a nearby station. As luck would have it, I had gone to cosmetology school with her three years earlier. I started there the next day. Soon my clientele began to increase, and my life began to become more stable. At last I was starting to mature.

CHAPTER 4

A TROUBLED
RELATIONSHIP

B y the time I was twenty-one, I was married and divorced. I never felt more free or alive. I instantly took my life back. I started my new job, met new people and for the first time in what seemed an eternity, was having fun! I enjoyed night life and dancing. I began to meet many enjoyable people and a number of men during this time. Between work and night life, food began to tumble down on my list of pleasures. I got thinner than I ever had been in my life. I rediscovered exercise—and a size nine! I took up bike riding as my form of exercise and hobby, and joined a health club in my area.

I had never been happier in my life. My good friend Mary Ann introduced me to a church she was attending, the Mile Hi Church of Religious Science in Denver. Almost immediately, I knew I was supposed to be there. The philosophy and way of life of Science of Mind was exactly what I needed at the time, and it began to influence me deeply. It seemed I could not get enough of it. I became a member of the Church and for the next two years enrolled in their Science of Mind courses of study.

At last, I was living the life I had always wanted and loving it! I had a great family and friends, and two great roommates, Wally and Stephen, who were like brothers to me. I
also was working at a job that I loved and attending a church
that taught me a sound, practical approach to living. I was
learning about spiritual strength. I was growing into an
awareness that God was always with me and in me, and I
knew I could always rely on that knowledge. I had an opti-
mistic and healthy outlook on life and looked forward to
every new day. In short, life was good.

During the next five years, I enjoyed relationships with a
few boyfriends and some casual dating. For the most part, I
dated really decent men with the exception of one—Mike,
whom I later discovered was alcoholic. I had met Mike
shortly after my divorce. We dated for about six months. I
watched him lose one job and demolish a car in only the first
month of our dating, and he was not even drinking then!
One night he was driving me home from the dentist when we
hit a patch of ice, causing him to lose control of my car and
crash into a road barrier. . There was considerable damage to
my nearly-new car, but no one was hurt. On the way home,
Mike stopped by a liquor store and bought a fifth of vodka.
That night he decided to go off the wagon.

During this time I still continued to go to church and go
out with my friends, although I knew I was being co-dependent to Mike's drinking. Eating had not remained an issue
with me because I was still enjoying a healthy lifestyle—with
the exception of Mike, who had resumed his drinking. I put
up with him for about two more months, until I just decided
the pain of the relationship was just too much, and I decided
I did not want him in my life anymore.

It came about when he asked me to pick him up from work one Saturday afternoon. On the way home he wanted to stop in a bar. I found myself next to him in a dark, dingy bar on a beautiful fall afternoon, wishing I were outside riding my bike. When Mike asked me if I could loan him five dollars for his bar bill (to add to the $600 he already owed me), I threw the money on the bar and walked out. That was the end of Mike.

Doing that was one of the hardest and most freeing things I ever did for myself. I walked away from a situation that did not serve me and could only pull me down. Even though it was not a healthy or positive relationship, I still felt a sense of loss and I grieved over its ending. I lost even more weight, and for the first time in my life I was into a size seven. I had no interest in eating. I sat at home and cried over my "loss." Of course, in a relatively short matter of time I recovered from this relationship and was soon enjoying life again and in a much healthier way.

Over the next few years, I dated a number of delightful and decent men. I was enjoying the fact that the opposite sex found me attractive. I confess that I felt some power in that. I wanted to date many different men, and I did. However, at some point in my life I knew I would want to settle down. However, this was furthest thing from my mind.

Until I met Steve, that is. Steve was the most decent, caring, and talented man I had ever known up to that time. He reeked of stability and loyalty. I liked him immediately, but I was not ready to get into a serious relationship again. However, he was persistent and charming, and I felt unable to resist him. I discovered we had much in common and, best of all, we truly liked one another. I was starting to plan my future with him.

My roommates Wally and Stephen liked Steve as well. Then, as quickly as he arrived in my life, he disappeared. I was confused and heartbroken. It was only later I surmised that the woman he had been dating earlier had become pregnant. I learned he accepted the child as his, and they married. Several months later I saw Steve and his wife with their new baby in a stroller. It was painful for me.

For the next several years I had fun dating different men and feeling good about my life. Food no longer seemed an obsession to me. Stephen and Wally were sane, sensible eaters. I baked quite a bit, mostly for the person I was dating at the time. Cheesecake, carrot cake, and mud pie were among my favorites. My roommates would share in these things and we seemed like a happy little family living in our big townhouse. Stephen and I would go on long bike rides together, and I played softball (quite badly) for Wally's team. In spite of the fact that my softball playing was not quite up to par, we did manage to win the division championship that year! I went to the athletic club three or four times a week to weight train and enjoyed biking when weather permitted. All in all I was having a good life. I was happy. Then I met Ron.

Ron was energetic, good-looking, held down a responsible job, owned a beautiful home, and was always willing to take a risk. We dated for several months. He had a rich sense of humor, though he could be quite sarcastic at times. He never let me pay for anything and was ambitious and active. Ah, yes, there was one minor detail I forgot to mention. He was married, which I learned only after we had dated for about three months.

I discovered it purely by accident. A client who frequented the salon where I worked had fallen into his trap earlier and dated him as well. However, it took her less time to "wise up." To say the least, I was devastated. I finally realized I needed to get tough and develop a backbone when it came to picking relationships. Instead of being addicted to food I was becoming addicted to destructive partners. Unfortunately, it took me another six months to separate myself from him and his overbearing personality.

My life and eating were beginning to spiral out of control. Our lease was up and Wally wanted to move on. I decided to get a little townhouse of my own so I could have more private time with Ron. This was all before I found out he was married. I gave my power to this man, and he abused it. It was while I was living by myself that I discovered Ron was married, and I did not have Steve and Wally around for support. So, once again, I turned to food for consolation.

Ron was compulsive in every area of his life—drugs, women, alcohol, you name it. During the six months in my attempts to drive him from my life, I gained thirty pounds. I was miserable with my weakness. I was overeating constantly and starting to feel isolated. One day I drove over to his house when I knew he was out of town. His wife Sandi answered the door. I told her everything. She didn't believe me. She thought I was making it all up. "Where do you think Ron was a few months back when he was gone several nights a week?" I asked her. Shocked, she said thought he was with his male friends.

I later found out Ron was a drug dealer and his wife, Sandi, who was also his secretary, was a cocaine addict. The whole situation was a mess. I needed a severe shock to change my life. Ironically, Ron provided it for me.

CHAPTER 5

A NEW RELATIONSHIP AND A NEW ME

Early one morning I received one of Ron's phone calls from yet another woman's hotel room. He asked me if I had time in my schedule that day to fit this woman in for a set of acrylic fingernails. Well, that cinched it for me. In no uncertain terms, I told him to leave me alone and never to darken my door again. The difference this time was that I meant it, and he knew I meant it. That same day I decided to not only get rid of Ron but thirty pounds as well. This I accomplished in a remarkably short period of time. I returned to my exercise program, which I had abandoned because of Ron. I also reduced my intake of calories. I joined a support group in Overeaters Anonymous and started attending my church on a more regular basis. I took my power back. Life was good once again.

A year later, while visiting a friend's home, I met someone I never expected to see again—Sandi, now Ron's ex-wife. Unexpectedly, she was quite pleasant to me. She said she had been free of cocaine for several months and had gained back some badly needed weight. We sat on bar stools at the kitchen counter, and she thanked me for "setting her straight" about

Ron. Sandi told me no one had ever been that honest with her before, and though she at first did not believe me, she sensed I was telling the truth. It was then she decided to stop her cocaine use and consider leaving Ron. I left my friend's home that night feeling gratified.

I feel I must state most emphatically that the twelve-step program is both a valuable gift and tool. Born into an alcoholic family, both of whose parents were involved in the program, I found myself naturally drawn to practice its precepts. I also discovered that the Science of Mind philosophy walked hand in hand with it. However, I must confess that though I met many wonderful people in OA, I failed to see any permanent or decisive recovery among its members. There seemed to be simple reason for this: I found it much more difficult to control the appetite by eating in limited quantities than to just quit eating those destructive foods all together. If food is our drug of choice, then like alcoholics or drug users, you simply stop using that "substance" which is causing you harm. Once you stop using it, no matter if it is food, alcohol or drugs, your mind is freer to start the recovery process. You have told your mind once and for all: "I am not going to drink or take drugs or overeat again!" Since we must all eat to maintain life, sensible eating habits require constant discipline. If not, the cycle of overeating will continue.

During this time of attending OA meetings and beginning my slimming process, I was contacting and dating some enjoyable fellows. One was an amateur pilot, Bill, who occasionally took me flying in a small plane he owned with a couple of others. Bill was a decent, stable man who treated me with respect. However, within days of my first date with Bill, I also met Rod. That was an experience!

One Friday night I went with a good friend of mine to a local nightclub. I happened to be wearing a new size-four outfit a co-worker had given me. I cannot tell you how thrilled I was to be able to wear a size four. I looked good and felt good when my friend and I went out that night. Several men had asked me to dance and I was having a great time. I finally took a break to recover my breath and visit with my friend. Then a waitress came over to me with a beautiful red rose in her hand. She pointed out to me a tall, handsome gentleman on the other side of the dance floor as the one who had sent it. I felt flattered and a little giddy. I walked across the room and thanked him. Rod was over six feet tall, with an athletic build, black hair, blue eyes; I discovered he was also quite funny. We were instantly attracted to each other, and Rod and I soon started dating. I was having the time of my life, dating two great fellows who were totally different from one another. Pretty soon I had to make a choice.

Bill and I went out a few more times, but my heart was with Rod. One day when Bill called to ask me out, I told him that I had met someone else around the same time I had met him, and I felt it just would not be right to keep dating him. To his credit, he accepted it gracefully and wished me luck.

During this time, my sister was getting married and, of course, I was her maid of honor. I was looking forward to the wedding, and I asked Rod if he would like to attend. It was an outdoor wedding on a beautiful summer day. Both the wedding and reception were a success. Rod was charming, and I was proud to have him as my escort.

A few weeks later Rod asked me to go to Boston with him to meet his father and stepmother. I found them to be enjoyable, gracious hosts. We stayed for three days. It was during this time that I discovered something about Rod that I found disturbing. He always wanted me to look perfect. He would monitor the food I ate and insist I get my daily allotment of exercise. When his father wanted to take a picture of me after coming back from a rainy early morning walk, Rod asked him to wait until I had showered and put on my makeup.

During our visit, Rod purchased two large bags of candy, but refused me any. He ate both of them himself in the three days. He then complained that he had gained five pounds on the trip! This kind of controlling action caused me to become more cautious about Rod. I began to keep a mental checklist on him, just as I am sure he was keeping on me.

When we returned from Boston, Rod introduced me to an aerobics class that he was taking a few times a week. In a short time I discovered how much fun it was, and I was hooked. I decided to take three classes that first week, and with the addition of my bike riding, walking, and weight training, and other exercises, I went from 126 pounds and a solid size four to 118 pounds and a size three. I lost eight pounds in one week just with the addition of aerobics classes. Well, that was all it took. I had reached my nirvana.

CHAPTER 6

CHANGES AND CHALLENGES

At this time in my life, exercise and food became my God. Though I was still dating Rod, I was becoming less enchanted with him. He wanted me to look thin and perfect at all times, yet still wanted me to go to dinner with him frequently and spend more time with him. This meant surrendering my exercise, which I was not willing to do. On the days I knew I would be seeing him, I would leave work early in order to finish my workout before we would go out. I would not eat all day and then sparingly with Rod.

I spent a lot of nights with Rod, but he never made overtures to me sexually. It was not part of our relationship. That issue was starting to bother me as well. I was truly beginning to feel that he just wanted a showpiece to date and control. Though we enjoyed each other's company to a degree, I found I wanted more out of the relationship. Unfortunately, during this time, I discovered that I craved something even more than Rod's approval—food. When I was alone, I started to binge on massive amounts of food. I would eat nothing during the day, exercise, then eat sparingly when I was with Rod. Needless to say, I was hungry all the time. So, I began to binge on the

nights we did not see one another. Instead of engaging in a
productive activity like reading or visiting with friends or family, I would eat. Then suffer pangs of regret and work out even
harder and longer the following day. This would become my
life for two full years.

I was now two months away from being twenty-seven. I
was living in a beautiful little townhouse and had acquired
another male roommate named Mike, who was a recovering
alcoholic. You might think we would have much in common
and be able to help one another; but that was not quite the
way it worked out.

We were both trapped in our private pain. Mike had met a
woman at one of his AA meetings and did exactly what AA
suggests you should never do your first year in the program—become involved with another AA member. He had
met her within weeks of joining AA and almost immediately
transferred his addiction to her. Though he was staying
sober, he was acting irrationally. Mike was paying his rent,
but he was hardly ever home. We were roommates for two
years, and I saw him perhaps for a total of three weeks. It
was quite unlike my other roommate situation. I had considered Stephen and Wally my friends. They provided me with
the pleasure of conversation and the security of companion-
ship. I was rapidly becoming disenchanted with Rod.

One night an important message came to me through a
dream. I have always listened with great attention to my
dreams. Obviously, not all of them bring messages, but the
powerful ones, the ones that I can recall vividly, are those
that I know I must learn from. This particular dream was
one of those. I dreamt that I was sleeping and then, in the
dream, woke up to see Rod standing at the end of my bed, as

good-looking a man as I had ever seen. I slowly crawled over to reach up to touch his face. As my fingers touched his forehead, I felt something not quite right, something that seemed like a mask. As I pulled at the mask, I was horrified to look at the face of a grotesque, disfigured human being.

I was so startled by the dream that I woke up. I knew then that I was being told something and decided to stop seeing Rod. I am sure it was a mutual decision on his part as well. Though he possessed a likable personality, I learned a number of disturbing things about him in the coming months. These included his increasing use of cocaine, as well as rumors of prostitutes and dishonest business dealings. My intuition seldom fails me, and it certainly did not in this case. Unfortunately, as my addiction increased I would attract more men with addictions of their own. It seems all too true that "like attracts like."

By this time, my funds were nearly exhausted. I missed a great deal of work because I needed to spend so much time exercising. I had always worked a nine a.m. to six p.m. day with a full clientele of great, wonderful women. Those with whom I worked were marvelous people who saw what I was doing to myself, but felt helpless to intervene to help with my addictive behavior.

A typical day for me was to get up around six-thirty and take an hour's walk. I would reach work by nine, work until only three, then arrive at the athletic club by three-thirty. I would ride the Lifecycle for an hour to burn off no less than nine hundred calories. I would then lift weights for about a half-an-hour, and finally take two aerobics classes back to back. I would usually leave the club around six-thirty or seven. I did this every day.

On Thursdays I had to work late. Because of the class scheduling, this permitted me to take only one aerobics class. I felt so unsettled and aggravated by this revision of my exercise program that I found myself becoming irritated with my clients if they were late and got in the way of my workout time. My obsession both with my craving for food and the exercise to offset the weight gained by my overeating was making my life miserable.

Needless to say, my income was suffering because I was losing about ninety dollars of work a day, and still spending money as I always had. In fact, more. Because I was feeling empty in so many ways, my walk-in closet was filled with clothes I seldom wore. The sizes ranged anywhere from size three to size ten. During this time I was still managing to fit into a size three. Even though I would binge on large amounts of food, I was smart enough to stay away from fats and sugars. I read every book there was to read about the fat and calorie content of foods. Five of them were my constant companions, which I consulted frequently.

During this time I also kept a journal to record not only my daily impressions and concerns but everything I ate and how much I exercised each day as well. I knew I was consumed by food and exercise; at the same time, I felt so self-righteous and "in control," that I was thoroughly convinced I could successfully condition my body to get it to look the way I had always wanted. I never looked anorexic, although I went through phases of that as well. I just looked thin, fit, and athletic. Following are some examples of my journal entries:

Friday, June 22

Thank you God for getting through this day without bingeing.

Item	Calories
English muffin	260
Soda	90
Two apples	180
Half orange	50
Total	**620**

	Calories Burned
1-hour walk	250
45-min. walk	200
30-min. bike	300
45-min. class	300
25-min. class	150
Total	**1,360**

Saturday, August 4

It was a "food day" today, God. Please keep me honest and sane. Tomorrow is a new day.

Item	Calories
Rice cake	50
Apple and oatmeal	120
Crackers	700
Shrimp	450
Stuffed halibut	350
Hush puppies	400
Spinach	100
Potato	150
Bread	200

Continued

Saturday, August 4, *continued*

Item	Calories
Ice cream	120
Brownie	250
Yogurt and bran cereal	500
Pecans	450
Malt Balls	400
English muffins	450
Misc.	300
Total	**4,990**

	Calories Burned
1-hour walk	250
20-min. bike	150
1-hour class	350
Leg workout w/weights	200
30-min. walk/run	150
Total	**1,100**

Monday, August 20

Thank you God for this new day. I stayed sane and had a terrific workout.

Item	Calories
Celery	30
Salad dressing	150
Two potatoes	250
Rice cakes	100
One-half banana	50
Two slices bread	200
Total	**780**

Monday, August 20, *continued*

	Calories Burned
75-min. walk	300
35-min. walk	120
40-min. bike	300
20-min. walk	75
Total weight workout	300
45-min. aerobics	300
30-min. racket ball	150
25-min. aerobics	50
Total	**1,595**

Friday, Sept 14

Keep me sane today God and do not let me binge.

Item	Calories
Slice of bread	80
Wine	300
Popcorn	400
Apple	90
Total	**870**

	Calories Burned
1-hour walk	250
20-min. walk	50
45-min. walk	200
40-min. bike	250
1-hour class	300
35-min. class	150
Weights	150
Total	**1,350**

Sunday, December 4

Total "blowout" today, God. I did nothing but eat. Too many calories to count.

	Calories Burned
1-hour walk/run	300
30-min. class	175
45-min. upper body weights	100
Misc. exercise	150
Total	**725**

Monday, December 5

Fresh start today, God. Keep me sane one minute at a time.

Item	Calories
One-half orange	40
Carrot	40
Two bites of bread	30
Three bites salad	30
Cabbage	20
Total	**160**

	Calories Burned
1-hour walk	250
45-min. class	300
Total	**550**

Too bloated to really work out hard.

As a rule, I did not accurately record my binges. It would have used up too much paper and ink! I just wrote it off as a bad day. Also, I am not sure whether my talking to God in my journal was all that honest. I knew I was slipping into a depression. Until I got help for that, my eating would remain out of control. I needed medication as well as prayer.

Rod was out of my life by now. I was immersed in working out, counting calories and feeling lost, obsessed and lonely. My depression seemed to be increasing.

One night my good friend Mary Ann gave a dinner party for the holidays. I was invited and, sensibly, brought a salad. I enjoyed good conversation with everyone, particularly with my old roommate, Wally, and many of Mary Ann's friends. Dinner was over, and I had eaten just enough. However, there was a great deal of food left over, so I started helping myself to seconds—and then thirds. Only this time I was not being selective about what I ate. I gorged on desserts, breads, baked beans—nearly everything that attracted my all-consuming appetite. I simply could not stop eating.

I finally left and went home. When I took my clothes off and looked at myself in the mirror, I was horrified. I had eaten until my stomach was so distended that I looked as if I were pregnant! I felt so miserable and uncomfortable, I wanted to cry. I had eaten to that point of excess only once before several years earlier. It had scared me then, and I was scared now.

CHAPTER 7

CONFRONTING MY DEMONS

The next day I continued to feel bloated, miserable, and hung over. My face was swollen from water retention. I did my morning walk as usual and stopped at the grocery store on the way to work. It was not to buy food, but Correctol laxative. Even here I was excessive and took ten capsules. I just wanted to rid myself of my feeling of bloatedness, hopefully all those excessive calories, and the misery caused by my stupid, undisciplined eating. After work I did my usual three-hour workout, but went home still feeling totally lost and out of control. I turned on the television in my bedroom, crawled into bed and prayed I could stay there until morning.

I did not eat for three days. I was feeling an increasing sense of isolation. Needless to say, I spent a considerable amount of time on the toilet for the couple of days following this incredible binge. I needed to drink gallons of water because of my thirst from all the salt intake, as well as the water loss from the laxatives. Unfortunately, this was not the last of such episodes. Others were to follow.

During the following months I dated at least four men at one time. They were all very cute. One of them, who worked at the athletic club, was particularly beautiful—and loads of fun. However, as I was shortly to learn, he really wanted a woman to take care of him, and I could sense that he wanted that person to be me. However, I was too smart and way too selfish to go down that road again. Another was a yuppie with a blossoming drug habit. The third one was a wonderful fellow who was desperate to get married. And finally, there was the successful guy who liked his women thin, very thin. I held on to him the longest. Eventually, he married the thin woman of his dreams shortly after we stopped dating. In short, during this period in my life I was definitely not interested in any kind of meaningful relationship. Dating was just another compulsion.

Oh yes, I nearly forgot one more—Steve, an alcoholic who, in spite of his problem, provided me with a great deal of fun and laughter. We adored each other for about a month. He thought I was beautiful; I thought he was successful. One night I made a great dinner for him, but he showed up ninety minutes late and drunk. That ended that relationship. I had enough problems of my own; the added burden of an alcoholic was too much to bear. I was coming to realize that my primary interest was my own addictions. Despite my best intentions, they were controlling my life.

Somewhere around this time I became amenorrheic—I stopped having periods. My body fat was only 9.5 percent. I knew what my body fat was, because I was compulsive about having it tested by anyone who knew how to measure it. I was seeing a nutritionist, not because I was really interested in learning about nutrition, but because I craved the attention. I wanted to be told how good I looked. Interestingly enough, should anyone mention even in passing that I worked out or exercised a lot, or asked why I didn't eat, I became exceedingly irritable. It seemed I talked about nothing but two things—the fat content in food and working out. I felt so self-righteous! How proud I was of the control I had over my 118-pound body. I felt disdain for people who were unable to resist a brownie or French fries.

What a boring, rigid, self-righteous person I had become! As I reflect on the person I was then, I do not find a very likeable woman. The holidays were a blur to me that year. I could not think of anything but food and exercise. My roommate Mike decided to move to the mountains and start a company. He was doing well and seemed happy. He was sober and feeling good about himself and decided to take a risk with this new adventure. I was truly happy for him, because he really was a wonderful person. I decided not to seek a new roommate. Most of my concerns centered around my obsessive exercise routine and buying new clothes on credit to fit my size three figure. Instead, I decided to further isolate myself and move halfway across town to live with my mother.

CHAPTER 8

EATING MY WAY
INTO MISERY

So, in with Mom I moved, and into the same tiny bedroom I had slept in when I was sixteen. I do not remember much about those few months, except that I still stayed
quite connected to the lifestyle I had been living. I tenaciously
held onto my exercise routine and worked only about thirty
hours a week. I still dated and still got further into debt. Instead of trying to pay off some of my bills, I seemed to spend
far more than I earned.

One beautiful Sunday afternoon I was at a local "watering
hole" with some of the people from the club where I exercised. We were enjoying each other's company around a large
table. Most were drinking beer. I was drinking water, of
course—beer had too many calories. Then one of the guys
mentioned he was looking for a couple of roommates. He
was just divorced, lived in a big house, and needed some help
in making the payments. So I soon had two new roommates,
Brad and Helen, and found myself living in a beautiful home.
I was looking forward to having roommates again. It felt
good to get my furniture back and be surrounded by my
things again. Since Brad did not have furniture at the time,

mine filled the living room perfectly. This could have been a great healing time in my life. Apparently, it was not to be.

Instead, the days and months to follow became a living nightmare of binges and purges and true insanity. Brad and Helen were sane, normal people—and sensible eaters. True, they occasionally partied too much for my tastes, but considering my own weaknesses, I was in no position to judge them. I am sure they knew what I was going through, but just did not know how to approach me on the subject. So, my problem was basically ignored, which suited me just fine. Or so I thought at the time. As soon as I moved in, I returned to my intense workout routine. An hour walk in the morning before work, at the club by three thirty for an hour on the lifecycle, then off to the weight room before doing my two back-to-back aerobic classes. All of this on a diet of maybe an apple, a couple of carrots, and a cup of coffee.

Well, needless to say, I was pretty hungry by the time my workout was over. So, it was all I could do to stay sane while trying to prepare my food for the evening. Many nights dinner consisted of two pieces of marinated chicken covered with onions and carrots and cooked in the microwave. Those were the sane nights. On the steadily increasing insane nights, I would drive to the grocery store after my workout, buy a box of raisin squares cereal, a box of bran cereal, a box of raisins, a few bananas, and a half-gallon of vanilla ice cream. I would blend it together in a mixing bowl and consume it all. Occasionally, I might leave a few raisins in the box and a banana.

As one might assume, the next morning I would feel drugged and bloated; my stomach would be horribly distended. I would then, as formerly, swallow a large number of laxative capsules and spend considerable time at work in the bathroom. After going to the bathroom, I would check my body in the mirror, feel for my hipbones and my ribs, waiting anxiously for the bloating to go away. There was not a time during those years that I did not look at my body in the mirror in detail every time I went to the bathroom. Am I still thin? Are my hipbones showing? Can I see my ribs? And on and on.

One summer night on my way home from working out, I again went to the store to get something for dinner. I felt I was in control, buying simply chicken and vegetables. However, I could not resist a box of Life cereal. On my way home, I found myself digging into the cereal, yet resisting the temptation to eat it all. I ate about a quarter of the box but, filled with a certain measure of guilt, tossed the rest out onto the street in handfuls.

My morning walk the next day was along the same streets where I threw the cereal. Upon reflection, I find it hard to imagine what I did next. I picked up the cereal that had been lying in the street all night, and crammed as much as I could into my mouth before I made my way back home. What a sight I must have been, picking up dew-covered cereal from the street at 6:30 in the morning! I can only imagine what someone might have thought of me if they had seen me doing that. Did I fail to mention my insane behavior?

During these months I dated several more men, still continuing with my compulsive tendencies. I confess I had little interest in most of the men I dated during this time. Their role was to provide me with a convenient diversion from my preferred obsession—food. I even dated someone I really did not like. He was in the Marines and I went out with him several times, met his parents, met his co-workers, all the while thinking "Why am I doing this to myself?" Again, another self-destructive, abusive pattern of behavior.

My Marine asked me to go on a weekend river raft trip with him down the Colorado River. I knew I never should have accepted the invitation, and later sorely regretted my decision. I had to stay the night at his house so we could get our early start. We left before dawn on Saturday morning to make it to our starting point in the mountains. Because I had done my usual three-hour workout the night before and ate next to nothing for dinner, I was already starving before we had begun. And I knew I could not binge in front of this super-disciplined Marine. We arrived at our starting point high up in the Rockies, and discovered I knew quite a few people on the trip. However, I found it hard to socialize. All I could think of was eating.

There is always the customary gorp on raft trips and bags of it were everywhere. Gorp is a snack food made up of nuts, raisins, chocolate chips or M&M's, cereal, and whatever else one's imagination dictates to toss in. I could focus on nothing else but the gorp.

People around me were laughing and having fun, and I was obsessed with the gorp. At the same time, I was developing an intense dislike for the Marine. We made it through the first day, which had been particularly beautiful, but I found myself unable to appreciate any of it.

The raft guides always make a great dinner for the people on the trip and this night was no exception. When we pulled out of the river and set up camp for the night, they filled huge Dutch ovens with lasagna, and then added salad and bread to the menu. Well, needless to say, I was primed for a binge. And binge I did. Not overtly, but I helped myself to at least six large helpings of lasagna and an entire loaf of bread. I also allowed myself some gorp. Not just some gorp, but handfuls and handfuls of it. I didn't do this in one sitting. I would fill up my plate and go off alone to eat. I would fill up my plate again and eat with some people, then go back to the tent and try to read. Reading would last for five minutes, then I would return, again fill up my plate, bring it back to the tent and eat.

Marine-man would then show up at the tent, and I would have to sneak out and find another place where I could take more food. This went on for about two hours. I know the guides were getting concerned because they are not supposed to eat until every one has finished They went ahead and ate anyway, probably for fear that I would eat it all! By the time I had finally finished eating, I again looked about six month's pregnant and was miserably uncomfortable. I finally crawled back into the tent and somehow managed to get some sleep.

Camp breaks early on raft trips, but there is also breakfast—eggs, bacon, and more bread. I had no interest in breakfast, and, of course, everyone kept asking why. That is always a question to place a binge eater in a decidedly bad mood. At this point, I had a T-shirt and shorts on over my swimsuit to cover my stomach, which was so distended. When it came time to put our life vests back on before getting back in the raft, mine would not fit anymore. I could not buckle it over my huge stomach. At this point, Marine-man, being somewhat confused about the whole thing, came to my rescue. As he reached to help me buckle the vest, I nearly bit his head off in front of everyone in the raft. I raved like a lunatic and certainly displayed some unladylike behavior.

I hated myself, I hated my body, I hated everything. By the time the day was over, I am sure I managed to alienate just about everyone around me. Marine-man and I headed for home, and on the way he stopped at a convenience store to get something to eat. Again, I bought Correctol and swallowed about twenty of them in the bathroom before we got back in his car. Oddly enough, Marine-man still wanted to continue to see me even after that miserable weekend. As a gift to both of us, I put an end to our dating after that raft trip from Hell. Many more men were to follow who were either battling addictions of their own or were nice, decent fellows. I rejected all of them, one by one.

Every time I would see Marine-man at the club, he would remind me that I still owed him $60 for the raft trip from Hell. I was out of control and so broke and that I could not pay him. I was too busy spending money on binge food or workout clothes. Finally, after about the tenth time of his reminding me, I told him I would pay him the following day.

When I got to the club the next day he was on the lifecycle, situated on the lower level. You could look down and talk to whoever was riding, which I had done many times. I leaned over the railing and told him I had his sixty dollars. Of course, he was happy about that. I then dropped sixty one-dollar bills on his head. Like green butterflies, the dollar bills floated everywhere. I must say, to his credit, he had a good sense of humor about the incident and laughed the whole time. Upon reflection, I believe he was really a fine person with great parents, a good education, and high goals, and was definitely on the way up in the Marines. All these things I know now to be true. But then I was in too much pain and too self-absorbed to be aware of any of it.

CHAPTER 9

MY INSANITY INCREASES

One summer night my roommates and I decided to host a party. Helen and I were discussing what kind of drinks and beer we would have, and when she said something about the food, I pleaded with her not to have any. Obviously, she thought I was insane. Of course, she was really unaware of my insanity and, not wanting to confess my obsession, I tried to offer rather pallid excuses.

"We can't have a party without food, Barb," Helen replied to my suggestion. "That's crazy."

"Why not? We'll just have drinks and beer. These people do not really need to have food around," I snapped back.

I was terrified at having enough food around the house to feed thirty or forty people. It was also incredibly selfish to expect these people to yield to my weakness, but that's how self-centered and selfish and out of touch my eating obsession had made me. I did manage to get through the party without eating, and I did have a good time when I was able to remove myself from thoughts of food.

By this time, my eating disorder clearly had control over my life. I was depressed, but failed to acknowledge it. I was unable to pass an entire night with uninterrupted sleep. I hated going to bed because I would wake up three or four hours later and pray not to get up and binge. At the time, I failed to realize that my inability to sleep through the night was a symptom of depression. I had no conception of just how devastating all the bingeing, over-exercising, and Correctol abuse was to my body chemistry.

I attended other parties, but my attention was always on the food. I recall one nice party in the late fall in which I noticed with obsessive delight a plentiful variety of hors d'oeuvres, food platters, and lots of desserts.

I remember taking a plate of brownies in the bathroom and eating them. Then I would take something else to the bathroom and eat it. One guest made a comment that I sure was spending a lot of time in the bathroom! It got to the point where I took Correctol with me everywhere I went, just in case I surrendered to that unexpected binge. This happened to be one such night. So I followed my brownies with the customary ten or twenty Correctol, and continued to hide out and eat secretly most of the evening.

The misery, lack of control, and hopelessness I felt during these binges are indescribable. There was never any joy or fun during a binge. It was just pain. Food can truly be enjoyable. It was for many years in my life. Now it brought me only fear and pain—the true meaning of addiction. Something that once brought me joy was now only introducing misery into my life. Yet I could not release myself from its grip. There was this huge thing missing in my life; it was called balance. Food and exercise were my only interest. How could I get that balance back?

The Thanksgiving holidays provided me with an answer. I decided to go to the Tucson Canyon Ranch, instead of spending it with my family. That way I would not be tempted to eat; I would spend all of my time exercising over the long weekend. So away I went, taking with me a girlfriend who had just had a baby. She needed to get rid of her baby fat.

So, off we went to beautiful Tucson on the Wednesday before Thanksgiving. It actually turned out to be a quite enjoyable time, because I was forced to turn over control of my food to other people, so I knew I could not binge. This had a tendency to reduce the power of the obsession, which was certainly much stronger when I was on my own.

I ate somewhat normally, though I exercised perhaps too much; however, that is what I went there to do. My friend had known for some time of my compulsive, addictive behavior. She thought it odd, but simply shrugged her shoulders at it. I am sure all of my friends and co-workers at the time knew how out of control I was, but felt either too embarrassed or helpless to confront me, thinking it would simply make me defensive and not do any real good. They would have been right. I knew I was sick, but I was not ready to do anything about it. I was also somewhat disappointed in my measurements taken for my fitness test: 33–26–33. Why wasn't my waist smaller?

The holidays came and went in a blur. There were many parties and many secret binges. I never felt at peace. Oh, how I wanted so much to be sane and happy again! I wanted to get a grip on my life but seemed helpless to do so. I even joined tried to join Weight Watchers, thinking that somehow I could turn control of my food intake over to them. The

lady at the front desk told me I was too thin to join. Of
course, I neglected to tell her how crazed and out of control
around food I was and simply wanted a little support with
my insanity. I turned around and walked out the door.

During this holiday season, I found myself moving into a
cute little apartment. Brad had a great new girlfriend who
had moved in a few months earlier, and I felt it was time to
move on. The insanity remained. By now I was twenty-eight
years old and barely able to make ends meet. I decided to
take a nighttime hostess job for extra money, hoping it
would again divert my attention away from food and exercise. It didn't work. Instead of doing something sane like
working more at doing nails and gathering up more clients,
I was scattering my energies even more.

While living those few months in that little apartment, I
met my next door neighbor. He was young (twenty) and
cute. He had a huge crush on me, and though I could have
easily taken advantage of it, I wisely decided to remain
friendly. At least I was smart enough in this instance not to
bring another person into my largely insane world.

This little adventure into independence did not last long,
and after six months I was back home again with Mom. This
time I moved my furniture into her garage. The insanity, of
course, had not left me. For the fourth time my younger
brother moved all my things. I am sure he was getting as
tired of my instability and weirdness as was the rest of the
family.

My tenth high school reunion was held that summer. I felt
like a total failure. I had just moved back home for the second time in two years. What a success story! I still managed
to have a few dates, but I was no longer hostessing and

working even less at manicuring. My clients could not handle the changes they found in my behavior, and many of them moved on to other shops. My life was on a downward spiral, and I felt that it was becoming the beginning of the end for me. My periods had resumed, and I remember how disappointed I was when it arrived after two years absence. That meant my body fat was no longer 9.5 percent. That meant I was losing the battle of keeping the weight off and that it was creeping back in spite of all my insane efforts to keep it off.

Depression was also beginning to establish its hold on me. I could no longer exercise, eat, shop, or purge my way out of it. I was feeling an intense sense of isolation and hopelessness, both of which I had created for myself. I was running back and forth to the other side of town to work and exercise and getting no joy out of either. I still did my three- to four- hour workouts, and I was struggling to maintain my weight; but the compulsive eating was starting to have its effect. At Mom's the food was much more plentiful than when I was living on my own or even with roommates. Mom shopped at the Army base commissary, and she purchased enough food for a month at a time. I could not leave the food alone. Knowing well my obsession, she even locked the extra freezer in the garage for fear I would get into the food stored there.

I was still not sleeping at night. I would wake at 2 a.m. with my heart pounding, desperately fighting off the desire to binge. Once in a while the temptation would be too great and I would give in, go upstairs and eat whatever I could find. Mostly it was either bread or cereal. I never knew which was worse, bingeing, or trying to fight off the need to eat. Either way, I was miserable. My anger was explosive and out of control, as well. I would lose it over the simplest things.

I remember the first time I moved back home. I was staying in my old bedroom, which was then the guest bedroom. When my mother had a friend visit for a few days, she stayed in that room and I moved downstairs. Before her friend arrived, my mother had rearranged the room to make it more comfortable for her friend. I threw a fit. What right had she to rearrange "my room" (that I was using rent-free, I might add)? Now I realize what an ungrateful "witch" I really was, failing to realize that I was even bingeing on her food for free as well!

I know now how out of control I was in every area of my life. And it was all because of this terrible disorder, which was causing such chaos within me. The nature of any disease is to survive. I was convinced my disease was firmly established within me, and I felt a terrible sense of helplessness to do anything about it.

CHAPTER 10

A Bout with Illness

Afew weeks into the fall season, a friend of mine asked me to house sit while she went on vacation. I was glad to do it just to have a change of scene. Oh, well, might as well binge in a different kitchen, I thought to myself. However, a couple of days before I was to move into her house, I began to feel under the weather with a sore throat and general fatigue. I went ahead anyway and moved to her house. I also looked forward to the move, for I would be close to the athletic club again. I did my usual workouts and went to her house and ate a great deal of whatever was in her kitchen. It was hard to get the food down because my throat kept getting worse; but even this discomfort did not stop my bingeing.

The next morning my throat was on fire. I went to the nearest walk-in medical clinic and waited to see a doctor. He seemed irritated that I was there. I got the distinct impression he was in a hurry to go to lunch with his nurse. He looked at my throat and gave me a strep test, took my temperature and said I probably had mononucleosis. He gave me a shot of penicillin and sent me on my way. I actually felt so bad I didn't work out, and the next morning I felt even worse. I called the clinic and told them I wasn't feeling any better and my throat was killing me. Their response was that it would take another twenty-four hours for the penicillin to take effect. I had experienced strep throat at least a dozen times in my life, and usually within hours of taking antibiotics I started to feel better. I knew I had strep throat, but the drugs were not helping.

The next morning, my mother called to see how I was feeling. I could barely talk; in fact, she could not understand what I was saying, my throat was so swollen and in pain. It happened to be my day off, so I drove back to the clinic and waited to see another doctor. This second doctor was great. He took one look at my throat and hurriedly excused himself. He was back in ten minutes and told me he had spent the last ten minutes on the phone seeking a specialist who could see me as soon as possible. He told me I was extremely sick, and that I had an abscess the size of a golf ball on my left tonsil. He said he could do nothing to help me because immediate surgery was required, and he seemed irritated that the doctor that had seen me forty-eight hours earlier had missed something so obvious.

Within half an hour I was in the exam room of an ENT specialist, who used a scalpel to drain the abscess. In a relatively calm voice, he told me I was about an hour away from suffocation. After undergoing a tonsillectomy, I remained in the hospital for five days. The day I was released I was told to take it easy and not do anything to raise my heart rate for eight days.

What do doctors know? The day I was released from the hospital I was at the club in an aerobics class and then did an hour on the lifecycle. I heeded no warning. The day I was put into the hospital I weighed 128 pounds. I lost a few pounds in the hospital and kept it off for just a few days, but then my old eating habits returned with a vengeance. I could swallow little else except ice cream and pudding for days. Believe me, I could abuse anything.

I continued to see the doctor for checkups in the days to follow. He continually stressed that I needed to let my body heal; and emphasized that I had been sick, very sick. Of course, I did not listen. I was still up to my same old tricks. He told me the likelihood of it happening in my other tonsil (only the left one was removed by the operation) was highly unlikely, but I needed to be aware of how my throat was feeling. Well, sure enough, four months later a slight infection began to develop on my other tonsil. I had to have that one removed as well.

When I went into the hospital for that surgery, I weighed 145 pounds. I had gained 17 pounds in four months! Quite painfully I learned that I could not out-exercise my binges. All the abuse I was doing to my body was taking its toll on my immune system.

After the second surgery, my doctor again emphasized that I had to let my body heal and perhaps I should reduce my exercise. Well, this time I listened to him. Not because I was concerned about my body healing, but because I was simply tired, tired of the struggle. I was already up to almost 150 pounds. Apparently, my working out was not helping much. So, in its place I continued to eat. I was almost beyond miserable. To make matters worse, I was down to working only twenty-eight hours a week.

Needless to say, my finances were a mess. Every credit card was nearly maxed out. Not only did I have car payments to make, but there were also payments on a piece of land in the mountains, where I hoped someday to build a cabin. The land was nearly paid for, but I was broke—financially, emotionally, and spiritually. I started to think about filing bankruptcy. Even thoughts of suicide were tugging at me.

However, before I took any action on either of these radical notions, I decided to spend down one of my many department store cards and purchase a Lifecycle imitation and replace my mother's refrigerator that was now on its last breath after thirty years of faithful service. I felt this was the least I could do since I had been abusing her hospitality for so many months and putting her through hell with my insanity. Buying the exercise bike was my last desperate effort to get control of my weight again, since I was no longer going to the club because of embarrassment over the weight I had gained. Gaining a great deal of weight in a few month's time is not the same as putting on the pounds over a period of years. Not in my case, anyway. My body had become puffier and more bloated because of the bingeing. My face was huge and swollen, and I prayed that I'd never see anyone from the club when I went to work.

When I was not working, which was increasingly common, I was sitting on the exercise bike watching daytime television. I then recalled that Oprah Winfrey had once been heavy but was now on a liquid diet and had slimmed down a great deal. Unfortunately, she was to regain all that weight and more in the months to come. I could totally relate to her and feel her pain, though I did not have to suffer her public exposure. My one, persistent worry was running into an old boyfriend or someone from the club. I had become such a permanent fixture at the club over the years that I sometimes replaced the instructors during aerobic classes. I am sure some of the women envied my perfect size-three body during those years. Indeed, some told me they did, but they were hardly aware of what I had to go through to get it that way.

On the other hand, I envied the women that lived sane lives and engaged in normal eating habits. I now know that many of the women working out at the club during those years had the same problem I had; I was simply not aware of it then. I often wondered why so many of them who possessed such cute little figures, size two and three, had such swollen-looking faces. In later months I was to discover that they were the ones who were purging through vomiting, and the reason their faces looked so wide, especially at the jaw line, was because the saliva glands had become swollen and distended by all that bingeing and purging. Swollen glands create a swollen face. I remember seeing a few pictures of myself when I was at my thinnest—and bingeing a lot. I always wondered why my face looked so fat. Bingeing was a good part of the reason. Although I could not get myself to purge through vomiting, (and I was grateful for this; it is a hard habit to break), I still overworked my saliva glands during a binge. Also, my face looked fat because of the bloating caused by ingesting a great deal of food in a short period of time.

CHAPTER 11

ON A
DOWNWARD SPIRAL

During this second live-in at home with Mom, I was hanging on by my fingernails. I was barely paying my bills, and now the bills from my two recent surgeries were starting to roll in. Even though I had insurance, the twenty percent portion I owed amounted to a few thousand dollars. I was not a happy girl. Then one night a friend asked me to go out. I decided to go, despite feeling miserable about my present condition. I had managed to lose a few pounds, so I was able to get into a pair of pants I had not been able to wear for a couple of months. This, at least, made me feel a little better.

We went to a local watering hole and spent some time drinking and dancing. One cute guy asked me to dance and then later asked for my phone number. He called me a few days later; we went out and I enjoyed his company. He did not seem to be bothered by the fact that I was living with my mother. He called me several times, and the next time we managed to hook up for a date. However, I had gained ten pounds since our previous date only two weeks earlier. I never heard from him again. I am sure he must have found my weight gain a bit of a shock. Also, my mental state was not all that agreeable. Why would he want to hang out with someone so miserable and so unpleasant?

More depression, more weight, more bingeing, and more depression continued. I know my mother must have been feeling frustrated and helpless. There is only so much a sane, healthy person can do for a sick, depressed and compulsive personality except to simply stand back and watch the insanity until it becomes impossible to withstand it. She had not reached that point yet; I still had to test her patience even further.

My bingeing on bran muffins is a good example. One day I went to the store as usual and purchased the ingredients needed to make them. Only I added something extra—a small box of my favorite laxative, Correctol. I ground up the little pink pills and added them to the batter before I baked the muffins. How clever of me! This way I did not have to take any Correctol afterward, and they would go through my system faster. This is a prime example of how sick my mind was at that time!

After I made the muffins and ate the first one, I realized that Correctol does not bake all that well, for when I bit into the muffins the taste of the little pink laxative pieces was disgusting. So I now found myself in a dilemma. I could not toss them into the trash because Mom would want to know why. I did not want to eat them, and I certainly did not want Mom to have one, because then she would wonder about that awful taste. Finally, Mom asked if she could have one of my muffins, but I told her they did not turn out very well and she probably would not like them. However, she insisted, so I let her eat one, praying the whole time she did not encounter a little pink chunk. After she ate the muffin, she said that she did not know what I was talking about; it was very good. How I prayed that she would not want any more. Happily, Mom never did encounter any of the bits of laxative. I do not remember what I ever did with those muffins, but I made sure she did not get another one!

More weight was starting to creep on. I completely stopped exercising, except for my morning walks, which were doing little for me because my eating was so out of control.

A very good friend of the family was getting married. We were all invited, but I did not want to go because I was getting so fat; also I had nothing to wear and no money to buy new clothes. The wedding was on a beautiful Sunday summer afternoon. Mom was gently prodding me to go. She went through her closet in a vain attempt to find me something to wear. However, I had made up mind to stay home— and that was that! She left the house all dressed up, looking forward to a happy occasion. I was feeling mildly depressed because I had refused to attend. In response to this, I decided to binge my way through the day. I made pancakes; not three or four, but ten or twelve, and ate them all with tons of butter and syrup. Then I binged on cereal and whatever else I could find. By the time she returned I had consumed at least 5000 calories. I am sure she knew I had binged, but at this point in my madness it seemed pointless to bring it up for discussion.

By this time it was mid-summer, and because of my financial woes, I decided to consult a bankruptcy attorney. He said my problem was pretty cut and dried; all I had to do was pay him $575 and we could petition the court for a Chapter 11 discharge. This meant I could keep my car and still pay on it, as well as keep one gas card. I think like attracts like, because when I met this attorney in his home, where he maintained his practice, I could not help but notice that it was filthy and disorganized. Though he was pleasant, he mumbled something about his son being in trouble for drugs and needing help. As I look back on this event, I recall how depressed and unhappy he was. It now seems only natural that he would attract me as one of his clients, who was similarly troubled. I paid him the money to file my Chapter 11. I felt bad about having to take this action, but apparently not bad enough to do something about my dysfunctional life and my severe eating problem. After a few months, my bankruptcy petition was filed in court.

So, here I was—a twenty-nine-year-old woman, living at home with my mother, having just signed papers to file bankruptcy and weighing well over 200 pounds. Actually, this figure was a close guess, because I did not really know my actual weight. I never weighed myself, fearful of knowing what the scales would reveal. Although the fact that I could not wear anything but a size 18 tent dress pretty much told me what I could not face.

The thought of suicide lay like a troubling alternative always in the back of my mind. It was not that I wanted to die; I simply wanted to end the pain that my obsession was creating in my life. At the time, I saw hardly any other options. The few days a week that I worked were extremely painful, as it must have been for my co-workers and clients. They would see me with my sad, swollen face, fatter than the day before, and wonder why I was torturing myself in this way.

Then one day my old roommate Stephen dropped in to say "hi" to me at work. He was shocked at how I looked. He had not seen me for several months, during which time I had gained more than fifty pounds. Stephen was always direct. He simply asked me point blank why I had gained so much weight. I shrugged and told him that "life has been difficult for me these past months." I am not sure that he was completely convinced of this answer.

My commute to work was about thirty minutes. During my drive I would give serious consideration to suicide and how to carry it out. Every time I made that drive I was either compulsively eating or thinking about killing myself. Oh, how I hated being me!

One summer day, Marilyn came over to my mother's house to talk with me. It was one of those days when I should have been working, but I had no clients booked for that day so I was in my mother's basement on a beautiful fall day watching Oprah and making a half-hearted attempt to ride my lifecycle. Marilyn asked me if I wanted to temporarily move in with her and her husband in an effort to try and turn my life around and curb my eating. She felt that living at home with Mom was too stifling. I might fare much better with them on their horse-boarding farm in the country, some twenty minutes away. I knew that I had nothing to lose by the change except, hopefully, overcoming my depression and getting a grip on my life.

The difficulty with any change of scene is that though it may change, the issues you are trying to escape from remain. You take your problems with you. So, in with Marilyn and Dan I moved. I tried to make myself as obscure as possible. Most of the time, I stayed in my bedroom on the lower level. I did my part in keeping the house clean, and I made a few meals now and again. At the time Marilyn was a flight attendant, and she was home only three or four days a week. So I spent a lot of time with Dan, which was not comfortable for either one of us. He had his own issues with anger and control and I could feel it, despite the fact I was so out of control myself. I did help him a lot out in the barn cleaning the horse stalls and occasionally feeding the horses. Dan was fond of guns and would take frequent target practice at the little prairie dogs around the farm. That always bothered me. I would see him abuse a barn cat or a horse, and it made me sick to my stomach. However, not enough to make me not want to eat. I could always do that!

During those months with my sister and Dan, I indulged myself in many binges. Marilyn and I had several talks about my failure to take hold of myself. She said that she was unable to notice any positive changes in my behavior. She was right, of course. As I suspected, a change in location did not seem to be helping.

In a lame attempt to gain control over my eating, I had a mouth guard attached to my back teeth. The purpose was to prevent me from opening my mouth more than the width of my finger, therefore making it extremely difficult to binge. The guard had two small balls that would fall between my back molars if my mouth was opened too wide, preventing me from being able to chew. I would have to push the balls out of the way with my finger until they sat on the outside of my teeth, permitting me to continue to chew. In order for the balls not to fall between my teeth, I had to take quite small bites of food. It was frustrating to eat this way, and it did slow me down considerably. It did not mean I ate less, however; it just took longer.

I cannot remember how I managed to pay for this contraption. I think at the time it cost somewhere around $500. I found a questionable dentist to install the device. I recall the dentist's office was quite dirty, and on first glance would be where no sane person would consider having their teeth worked on. However, we know I was far from sane at that time. When I talked with the guard in place, it sounded as though I had a big wad of gum in the corners of my mouth. Strangely enough, no one seemed to notice or question me on my new and weird way of speaking.

CHAPTER 12

ON THE ROAD TO
RECOVERY

Summer was nearly over, and my life with Marilyn and Dan had stretched into several months. Although I had been wearing my mouth guard for about two weeks, it seemed to have made little or no result in weight loss or intake of food. The thoughts of suicide seemed always with me. I hated myself, I hated Dan, I really hated my mother. I liked my sister, but I did not want to be around her. I did not want to be around anyone. The only thing I enjoyed in my life then was going down to the barn in the late day and feeding the barn cats. I spent what little money I had on cat food and, of course, food to satisfy my own enormous appetite. What a miserable existence!

One morning as I was I helping Dan clean out the horse stalls, I saw my mother's car pull into the long drive on the way to the house. I felt an instant hate and anger toward her. I really had no reason for these reactions, except for the fact that she was happy and sane and I was not. I was thinking to myself, "What does she want with (presumably) me at eight o'clock on a Monday morning? Can't she just get out of my life and leave me alone?" Well, I soon found out the reason for her visit. She had been calling various eating disorder clinics, located one in the area and wanted me to go there and receive the help that I needed.

My sister and she had obviously been concerned about my eating obsession and depression and carefully planned this little intervention. Of course, I instantly became defensive and strongly resisted the idea of going into a hospital for six weeks of treatment. What would I do about my car payment and insurance? What would I do with the few loyal clients I had left? Who would feed the barn cats? What would I do after I got out of the hospital?

Let us assess my adult life so far. A few years ago I was living with two great roommates in a beautifully furnished town-house. I had a wonderful job with a huge clientele of wonderful, prosperous women. I enjoyed dating and going out with my friends. I delighted in riding my bike and going to church on Sundays. I loved the classes I was taking once a week on metaphysical study. I had good, healthy relationships with my family and enjoyed spending time with them. I traveled to Mexico, San Francisco, Los Angeles, New York City, and Jamaica. I had a piece of land that was nearly paid for. I bought a new car every two years. I felt prosperous, and money was never a problem. I paid my bills responsibly and with ease. I skied every winter, hiked, biked and played softball in the summers. I liked my body and treated it well. I loved my town-house and enjoyed cleaning and decorating it. I attended many social events, such as fund-raisers, weddings of clients, art openings, and great Christmas parties. Perhaps even more importantly, I enjoyed food and ate sensibly and healthfully. In other words, I had a rich, full and balanced life.

Now what did I have? Ever-present thoughts of death. So, what did I have to lose? It did not take too long to convince me that I needed help. Of course, I knew something was terribly wrong with me, but I just did not know how to make the necessary changes in my life. When your mind is in a fog, it is hard to see what seems so clear to others.

It was decided that I would check into the Rader Institute for Eating Disorders. My mother agreed to take over my car payments, and my sister assumed my insurance premiums. For several weeks, perhaps months, I would have no income. However, they both felt that the financial sacrifice they were making was well worth it if, by doing so, it would straighten out my life.

The next day I drove to work, took care of the clients I had booked, and told them I was leaving to get some much-needed help. I gave my desk and my client list to one of my co-workers who had just started in the business and was trying to build a clientele. Although she was shocked to learn why I was leaving, she was both excited and grateful for the clients I turned over to her and for the head start in building her business.

CHAPTER 13

UNDER TREATMENT

On September 2, 1987, I was admitted to the Rader Institute, located on the seventh floor of a local hospital. The program consisted of six weeks of intensive counseling, therapy, and three monitored meals a day. No caffeine, no sugar, and no eating between meals were permitted. Time was intensely structured. My life was theirs for the next six weeks.

The first day was the intake, which involved weigh-in, photos, interviews with various counselors and doctors, and a psychiatric evaluation. I weighed in at 218 pounds, although that was never revealed to me because weight was not the issue; the reasons for eating were. I never learned my weight until I requested my hospital records for the purpose of this book.

The recommendations of the psychiatrist that evaluated me were as follows:

1. The patient should be engaged at the Rader Institute in all modalities of its treatment program;

2. The patient clearly requires antidepressant medicine;

3. Prescribe Elavil, which she has taken in the past with good effect.

Assessment: Clearly, the patient has an extremely marked case of bulimia and, secondarily, anorexia. However, she also has been significantly depressed off and on throughout most of her life. This is an interesting case in that her first major depressive episode occurred when she was eight years of age and led to the disordered eating pattern that has gotten the upper hand in her life.

Data: This is the first Behavioral Sciences hospitalization for this 29-year-old, white, single female. She has had problems with eating since she has been eight years old. She relates much of the reason for eating in a pathological fashion to the fact that she was depressed and also that her father was an alcoholic and was also doing something that was addictive. Colleague's notes describe the eating pattern that Barbara has developed. She has had moments of both bulimia and anorexia throughout her life. The patient, in taking a careful history, has had at least six major depressive disorders. Most recently, she has been depressed for the last two to three years. Her initial coping strategy for her depression was totally immersing herself in exercise. This woman would literally not only be working, but then would spend every waking hour exercising after work. She also became quite socially withdrawn when this depression hit her, whereas she described herself as a "social butterfly." The depression has escalated significantly in the last two months. She has been quite suicidal with strong ideation; however, no plan. She has almost all the classic signs of a major depressive disorder.

Mental Status Examination: Basically, the mental status examination was within normal limits, except for some of the depressive symptomology listed above.

So, they learned all that about me in my first two days. It would seem they had their work cut out for them! I was given a double room with a roommate. However, I barely got to know her since she was scheduled to be discharged in a week. However, in my first group meetings I learned that she was having a lesbian affair with one of the other women in treatment. The other woman had decided that she was no longer interested in men and "fell in love" with my current roommate. They did not seem to hide the relationship; in fact, they flaunted it. Although the counselors and administration frowned upon such activities, they could only control so much behavior.

There was also another beautiful woman in her late thirties and bulimic who was having a commonly known relationship with the only man in the program. He was in his early twenties, attractive, and had lost some 40 pounds. I could clearly see that many of these people were transferring their addictions from food to what I am sure were hastily formed relationships. I simply wanted to get better and get out of there. I had been down that same road before, of transferring my addiction to food to an addiction to a man, to exercise, to shopping or to some other destructive activity. Now I had a real opportunity to deal with the basic problem of my addictive/compulsive behavior and my extreme depression. I was not going to let it pass me by.

During the early part of my stay, while we were eating lunch, my counselor noticed me sticking my fingers in my mouth to push the mouth guard balls out of the way of my teeth. When she discovered it, she said it would have to be removed as soon as possible. Therefore, I made an appointment with my questionable dentist a few days later. My sister was good enough to pick me up and take me to my appointment. It was my first unsupervised outing in over a week, and it felt good. I certainly did not like being cooped up.

When we arrived at the dentist's office I noticed him sending some appreciative glances toward my sister. She was the attractive woman I had been, and I missed those complimentary stares! There was now an even stronger motivating force to get back on the road to recovery. Now with my mouth back to normal, I could hopefully start on the long journey to recovery. I had known what it felt like to be in love with life and to be happy. I wanted to be there again.

A typical day at the Institute was an early morning walk at 6:45 for fifty minutes or so, followed by breakfast, and then time for showering or other personal care. At nine, the real work began. The entire day was filled with group sessions with various counselors and therapists. At noon we had lunch. A couple of times each week, silence was required at lunch. The purpose was to concentrate on the food, feel a part of it, be aware of how it fills the stomach and nourishes the body rather than simply eating it quickly and unconsciously, and still wanting more. We took a full twenty minutes to eat, which meant we had to eat slowly and chew consciously. At the time those silent lunches were frustrating for me, as I am sure they were for most others, but I now see their purpose.

One day a week we attended eating recovery meetings, which consisted of a sandwich and a piece of fruit. The afternoons were filled with more group therapy and education about food and nutrition and eating. A few times a week we attended alcoholic recovery meetings held in the drug and alcohol addiction unit of the hospital. Alcoholics on the road to recovery were a little livelier than the food addicts, and I enjoyed the meetings. Perhaps I could relate to their problem, knowing I could easily have gone down that road too.

When I was in my early twenties and just after the end of my marriage, I was definitely into the party and disco scene of the early eighties. I could easily down ten to fifteen drinks (usually screwdrivers) in one night. I would dance and drink for hours several nights a week, not get home until midnight, then get up in the morning to do my hour walk and be at work by eight-thirty. I would work until six, run home and change clothes, then drink, dance and party all over again. Fortunately or unfortunately, depending on your viewpoint, I never had a hangover, no matter how much alcohol I consumed.

I knew enough about alcoholism to recognize that not having a hangover was not a good thing. Similar to my father, I had a high tolerance for alcohol. After months of drinking like that, I decided I could easily cross the line from heavy drinker to alcoholic. I did not want to go down that road, so I made a conscience choice to stop drinking for a while, and the biggest motivating factor was not because I did not want to become an alcoholic (although I certainly did not), but more because when I would drink heavily, I lost all my inhibitions and would end up sleeping with men that I had just met. Those were the days I would wake up and feel ashamed of my behavior; not because I drank too much, but because of my drinking I would have sex with someone I could care less about. I was lucky, however; many bad things could have happened to me during those wild months of partying that never did. I still loved to dance; so instead of alcohol I drank water, and I had a lot more fun. I also met a lot of interesting men that I eventually began to date on a more-or-less regular basis. I can drink now, but my tolerance for alcohol is much lower than it was then. My limit now is two glasses of wine. I have no desire to drink more than that, and I seldom drink more than a dozen times a year. I am grateful to be able to drink conservatively now.

Nights at the institute were for family counseling and guest speakers. Weekends were a little more relaxed; we had many outings to the zoo or hiking or shopping. I never really enjoyed the shopping excursions because I was so broke; I could barely pay attention, much less pay, for the fat clothes I did not want to wear anymore.

My mother was dedicated about attending the twice-weekly family counseling sessions. Her attendance helped me to work through the problems affecting our relationship. There I was able to release a lot of my anger in a safe environment. We were able to work through many of the resentments carried over from my childhood and teenage years. What were they? Now that I reflect on them, they seem obvious to me now! And they were even more so during treatment. For one thing, I remember my mom was seldom happy; she seemed always angry and stressed. She never demonstrated any nurturing or physical signs of love, such as a hug now and then. I never recall her ever saying that she loved me. It seemed to me that we children were simply a duty and a burden and raising us was certainly not something she enjoyed.

Now that I am an adult I can see why my mother was so resentful and angry. She had an alcoholic for a husband and seldom any money to feed her four children. It seems odd that I never felt anger toward my father, who was the primary cause of the problems we were experiencing and my mother's stress. Instead, I found myself blaming my mother for not leaving him. But if she did leave him, it would have

broken my heart, for he was my light. He showed me uncon-
ditional love, whether he was drinking or not. In my later,
teenage years, my mother grew much happier and we drew
closer, but oddly enough, I resented the fact that she seemed
so at peace. I felt she was somewhat self-righteous and un-
duly critical of me.

Family counseling lasted for another six weeks after treatment, so I am grateful to my mom for being there for me and
with me. After witnessing some of the painful relationships
many of the other women experienced with their families, I
really had little room to complain. Some of them had under-
gone emotional and sexual abuse, dysfunctional parents, and
generally bitter lives, which led them, in most cases, into
emotionally and physically abusive marriages.

CHAPTER 14

BEGINNING THE
HEALING PROCESS

By the beginning of the third week, I was starting to feel alive again. The antidepressants were starting to take effect. The Institute works hard those first couple of weeks to get you to the point of being emotionally naked. It takes about that long to break through some of the barriers we all create to protect ourselves. I remember one group session that was extremely painful. All my defenses were down; I was feeling exposed and "raw." However, I knew that was where I needed to be in order to begin the healing process. All my emotions were right on the surface, several years of bottled-up pain just sitting there, waiting to be released.

During this particular group session we were focusing on a woman who had entered the program about ten days after I arrived. I cannot remember her name, so I will call her Julie. Julie was a pleasant woman, who did not expect too much from life. However, she was holding in so much pain I do not know how she got through the day.

During one session, Julie started to tell her story of her eating disorder, of her bouts of compulsive eating throughout her teenage years. In her late teens she married her high school sweetheart, and they soon gave birth to a baby boy. She adored that child. However, her young husband turned out to have a severe drinking problem, and they divorced when the child was eighteen months old.

The custody agreement stated that the father could see their son on weekends provided he did not drink while he was with his son. Everything seemed to be going fine for the first six months. Julie said she was never totally comfortable in turning her son over to his father on weekends, but she had a measure of trust that he would follow the court order faithfully. Then one weekend when the father arrived to pick up his son, she felt particularly uncomfortable and ill at ease. Against her better judgment, she let her son go with his dad. The following morning, a policeman arrived at her door to tell her that her ex-husband had been in a drunk-driving accident and that their two-year-old son riding in the back seat of the car was killed.

During the telling of this tragic story, Julie never shed a tear. Nor had she ever shed a tear over her son's death, she told us. She said that such overwhelming guilt and pain were buried so deeply in her that they were unable to find expression in tears. The rest of us in the group, however, especially me, were all in tears. But Julie never cried, she said she could not, all she could do was to abuse her body with food. To some degree, we all felt Julie's pain. Perhaps in the telling of Julie's story, the rest of us were able to get in touch with our own pain and deal with it in ways appropriate to each of us. I experienced such unbelievable compassion and empathy for Julie, and also an incredible sense of gratitude that I was free of such a terrible emotional burden. I simply cannot imagine how I could have handled the grief and loss that Julie experienced. I wonder if this may be one of the many reasons I have chosen not to have children. I feel the loss of a child would be unbearable.

During this week my new roommate, Philomena, moved in. We hit it off immediately. I soon discovered we had a lot in common. She was fun and real and had the same intense love for animals that I did. Also we were both Irish. In fact, her aunt, who had come straight from Ireland, lived across the street from my mother's house. I learned that my mother was quite good friends with her aunt. Such a small world.

When Philomena arrived at the Rader Institute, she and her husband were living six hours away. It was a long trip for him to come to the twice-weekly night sessions but he continued to do so. Now, thirteen years later, Philomena and I are both living in the same small suburb of Denver less than two minutes from each other. We usually visit for a moment or two, when I pass her house on my bike and see her washing her car or watering her lawn.

When my husband and I were in Ireland a couple of years ago, he took some excellent pictures of the Cliffs of Moher. I left one of them on Philomena's patio as part of a big Christmas box that year. She said it "touched her heart." How lucky I was to make such a good friend in such an unexpected place.

There were also some incredibly fun moments during treatment. Sometimes during lunch or free time in the television room, something would strike some of us as humorous, and we would all laugh uproariously. I was finding out I could start to feel joy and laughter again. Those moments were always unexpected and welcome.

One Sunday afternoon we went on a day hike to a great little place that the counselor particularly liked and wanted to share with us. I loved every minute of being in the woods and experiencing the fresh air; at the same time I wished I were not so fat so I could move better and with more ease. When we got to our destination we stood around in a circle holding hands, and the counselor asked us to state one thing for which each of us was grateful. When my turn came, I said I was grateful to be able to feel the growing health of my body again, and to be aware that the numbness I had been experiencing was gone.

At the same time I still felt an incredible heaviness weighing me down. The carrying of seventy extra pounds was not only heavy on my body but heavy on my mind. I wanted the weight gone, and I knew with my sanity and self-esteem slowly returning the weight would eventually fall away. However, those of us with compulsive personalities want it done yesterday. I had to continually remind myself, "One day at a time." I developed a love-hate relationship with that saying for a considerable period of time.

Any treatment for an eating disorder is a day-to-day process. And it involves a lot of counseling and education about nutrition. I felt, at the time, that I could have taught some of the nutrition classes because of the compulsive manner in which I had studied foods—their calorie content, protein capacity, fat content and other nutritional data.

One day I was extremely anxious to get out and get going for our daily allotment of exercise. However, everything seemed disorganized. The person who was supposed to lead the group was late, so I became quite annoyed that our exercise time was being shortened by this person's tardiness. Later in the day, the counselor who led the session that morning told the rest of the staff that she felt I was too addicted to exercise; not only that, but I had a controlling personality. They felt it would be best if I did not exercise for a few days. They suggested I find something else to fill my time, perhaps reading or knitting. "I thought we were here to lose weight," I said. "You don't lose weight by not exercising!" They replied that I was not there to lose weight but to get my eating and compulsive behavior under control.

Obeying instructions like a dutiful inmate, I stayed in my room and wrote in my journal during exercise time. I wrote about everything that I ate during breakfast, lunch and dinner. My journal was not about how I felt about not exercising, but about what I ate and its calorie-fat-protein carbohydrate content.

A few days later, during one of our group sessions, the counselor asked me how I was doing with not exercising and what I was doing to fill the time, and I told her about my journal writing. I was instructed that I was still focusing too much on food and calories and exercise, and that I could not write in my journal anymore if the subject was simply about these topics. In other words, I had to redirect my life away from its obsession with food and exercise. For the first time I was presented with a real challenge to start to think beyond the two things that had controlled my life fully for more than two years. It was time to start letting go and growing up.

CHAPTER 15

STARTING A
NEW LIFE

I decided to just let myself "go with the flow" for the remaining few weeks and submit to whatever treatments the Institute felt best for my condition. One problem that the Institute did not directly address was constipation. Since my food intake was so drastically reduced, and we were not allowed coffee, which always helped me in the mornings, I had severe trouble with bowel movements. I was uncomfortable much of the time. Laxatives were out of the question because I had abused them so much in the past. In the nearly six weeks I was in treatment, I had only four bowel movements, and they were quite painful. The antidepressant I was taking also added to the problem of constipation. After my treatment I went to a clinic for a high colonic to rid myself of the waste that had accumulated over the weeks. It was a necessary, but not a pleasant, experience.

One of the patients was a cute college-age girl named Darla, who was at the Institute during the same six weeks I was. She was slim and athletic, with long, curly black hair. We all envied her figure. The reality was she had the same obsessive issues about food and eating as the rest of us; she simply did not let herself get fat. She chose to vomit to get rid of her excessive calorie intake. In a sense then, she had a different battle than the rest of us. Instead of having to lose weight, she had to learn how to maintain her weight by keeping her food down and treat her body with respect and kindness. A lesson we all had to learn in our own individual ways.

Darla also had other issues that involved men and addictions. She and her boyfriend had broken up a couple of times over the years. While she was in the clinic, they broke up again and it sent her into a tailspin. She wound up in a padded room in the mental health wing after a suicide attempt when he told her their relationship was finished for good. He came to visit her during her few days in the mental health wing. I got to meet him and he seemed to be a caring, sincere person. I am sure he must have finally tired of her dysfunctional behavior and of living with a woman with an eating disorder. They had dated all through college, but I assume he felt it was time to move on. I am sure he cared for her a great deal, but people who are mentally healthy can be driven away by those who are not.

Darla was cute and fun-loving and several men at the Institute tried to date her, but I am not sure whether or not she found anyone to heal her inner wounds. Perhaps a new relationship would have helped salvage her ego.

One Sunday afternoon my mother came to visit me. We were sitting at a picnic table on a beautiful fall day. Then she told me an old boyfriend of mine that had moved to Seattle had called to get in touch with me. Carl and I had dated on and off for about two years. He ended up working for my roommate, and we became close friends. He was younger than me and wanted to finish school. Meanwhile, I was on the fast track to destruction. I had then just started to date Ron (the married man—"Mr. Right"). Carl came back to Colorado to visit his family now and then, and we got together when he did.

I started to panic. I did not want to see Carl in my present condition, considering how I was looking and feeling. I wrote to him with some lame attempts at expressing the peace, joy and success I was experiencing in my life. Eventually, I wrote to him the truth of my real condition. He responded by wishing me well and promising to support my efforts to get well. We kept in contact through letters and occasional phone calls during my treatment and for several months afterwards. I also wrote short notes to caring clients who were both happy and relieved I was getting help. I eventually lost contact with many of them, but their notes to me were a great support at the time.

About the fourth week into treatment I was starting to get anxious. The antidepressants had definitely taken hold, and I was beginning to feel like my old self again. I just wanted to leave and get on with my life. I knew that I had to make a concentrated effort to lose the weight I was carrying and feel good about my body again. I realized I could not do it in treatment. I needed more exercise than a slow, forty-five-minute walk once a day. I have always been athletic, and I wanted to get back to a routine that suited my temperament. Biking is at the top of my list for exercise, and I yearned to get back into it soon.

Some of the women also were starting to get on my nerves. It seems they never sought to take control of their lives, but simply wanted to whine. Most had catered to their husbands or children and, unhappy with their back seat roles, began using food as a comfort blanket for their unhappiness. I must confess I had not gotten in touch with my compassionate side at this stage. But even now I despair at seeing women who choose to be powerless. Now that I was beginning to get my power back by emerging from my depression, I wanted to use that power. I wanted to truly "rejoin" my life and do something with it. The next week my wish was granted. It seems that my insurance could not be billed for the last week for some reason not known to me, so I departed at the close of five weeks instead of six.

Upon leaving I was at first shocked and even a little disappointed. Strangely enough, I discovered it easier to be impatient and anxious at the Institute, than to live in the outside world again. Fortunately, that feeling did not last long; I soon found myself looking forward to reentry. I knew I had to start my life over again, find a job and a place to live. I was also dead broke.

I found myself living with Marilyn and Dan again, but I promised myself it would only be until I could figure out what I was doing with my life. It was the middle of November and I went to work with my good friend, Mary Ann, at a salon where she was employed. Many of my former clients were now having their nails done by one of the manicurists who worked there. However, I never felt quite right working there. I seemed to be out of my element. I also knew I had to start building my clientele again. My new co-workers were sending me a few clients, but it was slow going. The owner of the salon was a man in his mid-forties, who had a surprising fondness for heavy women. I found myself still very much in that category. He indicated he wanted to help me professionally and, from what I could gather, woo me as well. I was still feeling uncomfortable about my appearance, so his attention did flatter me. At any other time in my life, I would never have given his attention a second thought.

One day during the December rush that every salon experiences, I was waiting in the reception area in between the very few clients I had, when one of my former clients entered. When I addressed her by name, she looked confused and did not seem to recognize me. When I told her I was the manicurist that used to do her nails a couple of years before, she looked at me with disapproving eyes and said, "My, I hardly recognized you. You have gotten so heavy. How much weight have you gained?"

Yes, that encounter nearly reduced my self-esteem to zero. Even though I had been seriously depressed, suicide never entered my thinking during the period of my recovery. However, I was far removed from the happy and self-confident person I had been just a few years earlier. I knew I still had a long way to go to get there. I was still wearing only my fat clothes, sizes 18 and 20, and I had no money to buy any new ones. In any case, I refused to buy any more fat clothes. I wore the same two or three things over and over—a big purple sweater over XL leggings, an equally large white sweater over XL leggings, or the purple sweater over my size 20 sun dress that I had first worn when I entered the Rader Institute.

To bring me what he thought would be some pleasure to the holiday season, Carl called to announce he was in town to see his family and asked if we could get together. This wasn't exactly what I needed to cheer me up since I knew there would be more than just the two of us. He wanted to introduce me to his "cute, funny" new girlfriend he had met on campus. When I heard this news, I wanted to dig a very large hole (because that is what it would take to fit my big body in) and crawl into it. In my fantasy, when I emerged I would be the thin person I used to be.

Carl and I were to meet for drinks, at which time I would meet the new girlfriend. Luck was on my side that particular day, because we had an incredibly bad snow storm, and we both decided it was not worth driving fifteen miles each way in such bad weather. How grateful I was for that snow! As it turned out, we never did see each other that holiday season.

That Christmas my brother gave my mother a kitten. Since she was allergic to it, it became another member of the barn cat community at Marilyn and Dan's. I felt sorry for the little guy out there on his own in the cold, not big enough to fight for his food—or even catch a mouse. So, I went to the barn every day to feed him. However, he was not adjusting too well to his new environment. By the end of January he was terrified of everything but me. Dan had decided to put him up in the rafters of the barn to keep him a little warmer, but it was incredibly cold that year. On January thirty-first (just after the Broncos took a hellish beating at the Super Bowl), I went out to the barn, pulled him down from the rafters and kept him secretly hidden in my bedroom. Dan forbade any animals in the house, still another reason for my dislike of the fellow.

CHAPTER 16

NEW EMPLOYMENT

Soon after this experience, Dan asked me to move out of the house. This was an unbidden gift. I needed to move on, and it was just the motivation I required—even if it was an unpleasant one. I then decided to stop doing nails altogether. I was able to secure a school loan and enrolled in a school for court reporting. My mother was quite proud of my decision to find another trade and gain more education. To support myself, I delivered pizzas at night and went to school during the day. I did not give up my nail business altogether. On weekends I would make house calls to some of my loyal clients' homes and do their nails. However, I was barely making ends meet. I moved into a basement apartment in north Denver fairly close to the school and with my new kitty (Theo). I put my nose to the grindstone. How nice it would have been to put that "grindstone" to other parts of my body! When I was fitted for my pizza delivering uniform, they could not find pants big enough to fit me; they had to be tailor made. I drove down to East Colfax, a somewhat unsavory part of town, to have them fitted. When he took my measurements, the tailor simply shook his head, muttering that it was too bad I was "such a big girl."

How I hated delivering pizzas! I also disliked school, but I was determined to stick it out. Then I had a stroke of good fortune. A friend of mine was working at Supercuts hair salon. They had a position available that would nicely feather in with my school schedule. So I happily quit delivering pizzas and started cutting hair. Actually, the money was not any greater; it was just a better job in a better part of town.

My apartment was small but comfortable and attractive, because I had made an investment in good furniture in former years, when I had sanity and money. I loved my little Theo; we were a team. I so looked forward to coming home to him at night. He was my first true commitment. I was almost thirty years old, and I had at last fallen in love—with my cat.

It was right around this time that Marilyn came over to my little basement apartment to tell me she was leaving her husband. They had both decided to quit drinking when they married, because drinking had been a serious problem for both of them. Marilyn sincerely quit, but Dan started again about a year into their marriage. He managed to keep it largely hidden from her, since Marilyn was gone much of the time because of her job as flight attendant. The secret was out when she returned unexceptedly one night only to greet Dan four hours later, who arrived home drunk as a skunk. I am sure because he had to hide his addiction for such a long time and felt guilty about it, he turned into such an unpleasant person. I could certainly relate to his mental state, though I could not forgive his callousness toward animals and his treatment of my sister.

I was now working hard at getting rid of my excessive weight. I knew I needed quite a bit of exercise, but my schedule did not allow for as much as I would have preferred. The antidepressants I took did not help. The one I was using kept me constipated and made losing weight difficult. However, I was not one to surrender. In the mornings I would get up and take a power walk before school. Then, after school, I would go right to work and sometimes get in another quick walk before my shift started. Sometimes I would not walk in the mornings because it was not totally light, and the neighborhood was not safe. Several times spooky characters that lived in the area would follow me. As an alternative, I would try to get in a good bike ride between school and work. Even then weird men would yell at me as rode by. I never felt safe or comfortable in that neighborhood, but it was all I could afford at the time.

School was not all that easy for me. The basic academic requirements as well as the legal aspects were far easier to learn than the steno machine with its peculiar language. In order for me to become skilled using the machine, I needed to practice for at least two hours a day. Usually I was home by nine-thirty each night, and then two hours of practice before bed. In addition to this, I had to study for the academic tests as well.

During this time, my car was broken into twice while it was parked behind my apartment. My apartment was burglarized as well. The thieves stole my few good pieces of jewelry. What bothered me the most was that Theo was terrorized while these men (I assume it was more than one, considering the damage they did) ransacked my apartment and trashed the place. I had gotten a new little kitten just two weeks before. He was at the vet's office getting neutered on the day of the burglary. As luck would have it, I had taken the money out of my top drawer to pay the vet bill before I dropped the kitten (Bootsley) off. At least that expense was saved.

I found out weeks later that the guys who broke into my apartment were looking for someone who had lived there two years earlier. Apparently, the fellow still owed them some drug money, and they had taken a bus from California to collect their debt. Obviously, the robbers were not overly bright. One look at my incredibly clean, decorated apartment containing nothing but female clothes should have told them their erstwhile friend had split. Not wanting to make the trip from the West Coast without some profit, I am sure they then decided to ransack my apartment.

Obviously, this was not the best of living conditions. My apartment was in a questionable part of town, just two blocks away from a halfway house for mentally troubled men. I began to feel stressed and unsafe living there and began to have nightmares about being broken into again. It was becoming even harder for me to focus on studying, not to mention that I was not having much of a love affair with school.

After four months, I decided to quit school and work full time at Supercuts. This was a huge relief to my mind and soul. Although on some level I felt guilty about quitting, I reasoned that if I hated school this much, how I could I possibly be a success in the field for which I was training? I did not want to do something I dreaded for the rest of my life.

Carl and I had been keeping in touch on a regular basis. He was currently in between girlfriends and his brother was getting married here in Denver. Carl and I decided he would stay with me for the few days he was in town for the wedding. He invited me to be his date for the event. It was something for me to look forward to in order to get motivated to shed a few more pounds. By this time, I was a solid size 16. Though I never weighed myself, I must have dropped about thirty pounds since leaving the Rader Institute.

I had mixed feelings about seeing Carl. The last time he had seen me I was a size four and weighed 122 pounds. It would certainly be a shock for him to see me so large. My hair was also quite long. I am sure I looked nothing like what he remembered. We had also made plans for me to come to Seattle to visit him on my vacation, which was a couple of months after the wedding. All these plans were made over the phone and through letters. My concern was he would not want me to visit him when he saw me after so many years. As it turned out, my concerns were unfounded—although there was some shock on Carl's part. He just kept looking at me, saying that I looked so different.

The wedding was fun. Carl and I enjoyed one another's company, though he remained busy seeing old friends and family. We really did not spend much time together. It was a very fast weekend and over quickly. I felt edgy and a little disappointed when he left. Something was not right, but I was unable to determine where the fault lay. My tickets to Seattle were booked and paid for (with the insurance money from the break in). I was uncertain if I should still go, but I decided to wait and see Carl's reactions the next time I heard from him.

I talked with him several times before my trip to the Northwest, and there seemed to be nothing in the way of my making the trip. I did go, and we had an enjoyable time; but something seemed wrong. I got the distinct feeling he was involved with someone else. He was also very busy with work and school, and I know it was pressing for him to take time away to entertain me. And I was certainly different from the person he knew years earlier. I was self-conscious because of my weight and insecure about my future. I also felt guilty about quitting school. Even though Carl suggested I move to Seattle and get a job cutting hair, I knew he did not mean it. So, at the end of my trip, he drove me to the airport, gave me a hug, kissed the top of my head, and that was the last time I was to see him. We wrote to each other a couple of times afterward, but we both knew it was a waste of time. I felt sad and rejected, for he was an important part of my past. Was I being told it was time to move on?

During this same period, I reconnected with Dan, another fellow I dated during the same time I knew Carl years earlier. Dan was decidedly good for my ego. When he saw me, he told me how beautiful I looked, and how much he liked my long hair. I always liked him, for he was always a lot of fun; but, again, he was a part of the old me. Dan I went out several times after I got back from Seattle, but the relationship fizzled. I knew it was time to get to know myself better by being by myself. This would begin a five-year period of relative isolation, in which I would begin a long process of reintegration.

I decided to get back into doing nails and landed a great job with a terrific little salon in Boulder. I was busy from the moment I walked in the door, and loving it. I was making good money again and liking the people with whom I worked. It was there I made some really great friends that I still retain to this day. I decided to move closer to work and found a beautiful little duplex not too far from my mother's house. I adored that place, and I was so happy with my job.

I was feeling alive again and grateful for my new life. I was down to a size 14 and still working hard to get rid of the rest of my excess weight. I had weaned myself off the antidepressants and the pounds were coming off a little easier now. Life was becoming good again. Every morning I would wake up in my perfect little house and thank God for the blessings I had received. I had two wonderful landlords that lived next to me in the other half of the duplex, and they could not have been more accommodating or gracious.

I also acquired another cat, Gray, who had come to my front porch one day and would not leave. After some thought I decided to keep him, but he needed to be neutered and given his shots as he was to become an indoor cat. Apparently, his wandering days were not over, for he did not come home the night before we were to go the vet's (typical male!), but he arrived again the next day and into the vet he went. Gray hasn't wanted to leave since. He likes getting fed on a regular basis and not being engaged in a cat fight several times a week.

I was now beginning to fear that I was going to become like one of those spinster women living in a house crawling with cats. Therefore, I swore off any more animals. Instead, I volunteered at the local humane society one afternoon a week. I not only enjoyed my work with the wild animals, but I learned a lot about them. They decided to place me in the wildlife section, feeding the raccoons, rabbits, wild birds, foxes, and others. I loved doing this. I can now appreciate why so many people can love animals the way I do and devote their lives to their care. It felt so good to be active and productive again.

CHAPTER 17

LIFE STARTS TO
LOOK UP

I met a good-natured co-worker at the salon. However, every day that I worked with this person, she complained about the extra five pounds she was carrying, and how much she hated her big stomach. Apparently, that was where her five pounds were living. I was forced to hear about what she ate the night before, and what she was planning on eating that day, and a great deal about fat and calories. Sheri was 22 years old, and all she could think about the majority of the day was her five pounds, and the food that was the culprit in creating them. Well, I thought to myself, I am getting paid back for all my early obsessive behavior by being forced to listen to her problems that were so closely parallel to mine. I guess I deserved that.

I was also grateful that this issue was getting further away from my life now and receding into past memory. One day, after listening to her endless complaining, I lost my patience and told her: "Sheri, there are bigger things in this world to worry about than your five pounds. Can't you concern yourself with something other than your weight and food?" At first she seemed a little shocked, but agreed that she needed to think about something else. God provided it for her. A few weeks later her father became critically burned when his house caught on fire. After three weeks of intense suffering in the hospital, he died. Suddenly those five pounds and what she was eating did not seem so important to Sheri. That incredibly tragic event was a wake-up call to her to live in the moment and refuse to be so self-obsessed.

About eight months into my new job, the owner decided to sell her business. The new owner was wonderful, and we all loved her. I had a constant smile on my face. I had a great job with a fabulous new boss, I played with animals once a week, I lived in a cute little house, and I was finally shedding some pounds. I was content.

It was then I decided to take scuba lessons—and a vacation. Our new boss had offered vacation pay after a year of employment (unheard of in this business). I took a couple of weekends off and did an intensive scuba certification. Then I put a deposit down on a six-day dive trip to the Bahamas, about four months away. I was really excited. It would be my first paid vacation doing something I had always wanted to do. I would live on a sailboat with twenty strangers and scuba dive every day. It was an adventure of a lifetime—well, my lifetime, anyway.

Then an unexpected event occurred which would turn everything topsy-turvy. For nearly a year now, my life had been proceeding smoothly. My trip was scheduled for late April, and I was looking eagerly toward it. Then late in the evening I was awakened by a phone call from one of my former co-workers, M., who informed me that the present owner of the salon had run into financial trouble. The former owner was going to take it back. While all this was taking place, the business was to be closed down for a period of time. Even worse, none us liked or wanted to work for that owner again. Overnight I was out of a job. I was also to discover the next day that my last paycheck had bounced. Goodbye paid vacation and happy little salon.

M. and I discussed our situation. We decided that since we shared so many of the same clients, it would be a good idea if we tried to land in the same salon. M. did skin care for the same salon I had formerly worked in, and we had started within weeks of each other. After an energetic search, we found a salon that would accommodate both of us. Since we shared so many clients, it only made sense to find a place to work that could accommodate both of us. The owner of the little nail boutique was most gracious and willing to help us in any way she could. There was a small skin care room available for M., and they made a space for my little manicuring table. We were back in business. We put an ad in the local paper and sent out cards to let clients know where to contact us. We had to scramble for a few days, but our clients were wonderful and happy that we were still performing our services. Our previous salon was still closed and never reopened.

While all of this stress was going on, I could have easily binged, as I would have done in former years, but I did not. The thought never occurred to me. I had just wanted to find another place to work. It was a tough first couple of weeks, but I got through it. At this stage in my life, the only role food played in my life was to satisfy my hunger (now under control) and nothing more. I had at last recovered my sanity around food. An employment crisis created the test for me, and I had passed it with flying colors.

It did not take long for M. and me to come to the conclu-
sion that we should open a business of our own. The main
problem confronting us was that I had no credit because of
my bankruptcy and M.'s credit was questionable. Then her
marriage to a wonderful husband came to our rescue. He let
us use their house as collateral on a commercial lease, and I
was able to borrow money from my mother. Off we went to
start our own little skin care, body care, and nail care salon.
It was the worst and most costly mistake I ever made. The
mistake was not because of my lack of good business sense,
I just did not have good business-partner sense. Although I
never obtained a formal degree in business administration,
the two and a half years we were in business together certainly earned me the equivalent of one. Even so, I was not
smart or perhaps educated enough to notice all the little red
flags that kept popping up to warn me about my future partner. But for the moment, the future looked bright and our
spirits were high. Only later would the clouds of our partnership start to darken.

It took M. and me a few months more to get our newly
leased space ready to open; in the meantime, I decided to go
on my dive vacation. At this point, with all the excitement
and stress involved in starting a business, I felt some hesita-
tion about going. But it was either go or lose my $1,200 ad-
vance payment on the trip, so off I went to the Bahamas. It
was the best trip of my life. I had nothing but fun. I met some
great people, and my ego was boosted by the attention given
me by a couple of single men on the boat. I developed a
crush on one of them; the other had a crush on me. It was
harmless fun. We played and partied and dived for six days.
The weather was perfect, the food was delicious, and the

company of twenty people I grew to know was equally wonderful. I lost about seven pounds on that trip. Scuba diving is a great way to burn calories!

I found I could not get enough to eat (though not by my earlier standards!). Being in the water three hours a day really makes one famished. I was still chunky, but I made the decision to not worry about it on the trip. I was about a size 12 and around 165 pounds. I could hardly wait until I was a size 8 to start living my life again. I did feel somewhat self-conscious in a swimsuit , but I quickly got over it. Nobody seemed to care. Like me, they were there to dive and relax, not to analyze my body.

After returning from my trip I felt truly alive! I was excited about my new business and happy with myself that I could take a vacation alone and have a great time. It was then I decided that I could be happily single for the rest of my life. I took a risk, I did something I wanted to do, scuba, and I traveled by myself. Now I was opening my own business. I am sure these are things people do all the time, but it was a big accomplishment for me. I felt good about myself, with a bigger and more genuine sense of confidence.

I continued to lose weight, mostly from the stress of putting a business together and from a couple of red flags that went up in my stomach from interactions with my future partner. I have learned to pay close attention to those feelings in my stomach. When all facts and figures fail me, I can always count on my gut feelings. Unfortunately, I did not take heed of those red flags in my experience with M. That was to be my biggest lesson learned—as well as dozens of others.

A few weeks after my vacation, I was told of a friend's approaching birthday. She and another friend convinced me to go out and celebrate. I really did not want to go out. It had been a busy week, and M. and I were busy putting our business together. We were meeting with various leasing agents and attorneys just about every night after work. However, I finally relented and decided to go out with my two friends, but only on the condition that we would go to the nightclub where my younger brother worked as a doorman.

As it turned out, my brother was not working that night. However, I did meet someone that night who would play a far greater role in my life. Kevin was handsome, and I felt attracted to him. We danced a few times, and he asked for my phone number. With some reluctance I gave it to him, for I was now quite cautious with any new man to whom I was introduced. Too many nightclub scenes in my twenties were still fresh in my memory! However, I had quite a different feeling about Kevin. Although I was sure I would hear from him, and I was certainly attracted to him, I was not at all sure I wanted to involve myself in another relationship after enjoying several years of single life. Was Kevin going to turn my life in a different direction?

CHAPTER 18

A NEW AND LASTING
RELATIONSHIP

Kevin and I talked on the phone several times before we actually went out. We soon discovered we had a great deal in common and shared a lot of laughter over the phone. One major problem faced us: we lived ninety miles apart! It was starting to literally become a long-distance relationship.

There was one thing that even distance could not prevent. I knew, even before our first date, that we would marry. When we started to see one another regularly, I found myself feeling calm and serene in his presence. Anxiety and doubt never raised their ugly heads. I had that good old gut feeling that he was the right guy for me. (I was smart enough not to tell him that until after we were married for a couple of years!) Heeding that feeling was a good test of my will to trust my inner self. It was also the first time I had ever felt that way about someone I was dating. I knew that deep feeling was necessary in order for a relationship to really work, and ours did! When I feel such peace, I know I am making the right decision. Those often painful years I spent in getting to know myself helped immensely in their own odd way by rewarding me with this relationship.

Kevin and I soon began to spend our weekends together. During the week I worked hard at serving my clients and preparing my new business for opening day. Many nights were devoted to shopping for equipment, linens and other furnishings for our salon. We finally opened for business in the middle of August. Kevin became an invaluable help during the moving process. He put together many pieces of equipment for us, wired our stereo system, hung mirrors and doors, and did just about anything else we needed done.

My mother and sister were there as well, unpacking linens and other things, helping to hang pictures and do other necessary tasks. M's husband was out of town; however, she finally showed up one afternoon with a cappuccino for herself and unnecessary office supplies. I was beginning to do a slow inner burn. It was then (knowing I had my name on a five-year lease) that I realized that this business partnership was going to have problems.

I was thinner than I had been in years. Though I was into a size ten, that pleasure was to a great extent offset by the strain of existing in a dysfunctional relationship. M. and I were only a few months into our venture, and yet I found myself feeling so much resentment toward her that I found it difficult to be happy about our new, thriving business. Since I did not have any productive release for my anger (Kevin and I were still seeing each other only on weekends), I felt myself starting to slip into some minor binges. Fortunately, they remained only temporary temptations, and the urge to eat excessively as I had in earlier years did not overtake me.

I still exercised every day, loved my clients, and visited with my family; but I did not inform anyone about my negative feelings. This was partly because I was embarrassed over being taken advantage of by M. and showing such poor judgment of character. The truth is, early on I had a gut feeling about her; unfortunately, I did not obey it. I had experienced her charming ways, and was suspicious of them, but chose to ignore these signals for the sake of the business. Again, I was selecting anger and food over God and inner direction. I needed to start meditating again and seek guidance, because I knew this situation was moving beyond my capacity to control it.

For the moment, I decided to lose myself in work. I hired someone to help generate more income and hoped for the best. M. and I seemed to get along fine on the surface, but deep down I mistrusted her. She was artificial and self-centered. In order to combat my growing irritation and anger, I found myself bingeing, usually after I would leave Kevin on Sunday, and sometimes during the week. However, these binges were not nearly so extreme as in former years. I certainly did not want to return to my earlier periods of depression and insanity. I turned to God more and asked for help. I was diligent about praying and being grateful, regardless of the conflict with M. At times, I felt I was hanging on by my fingernails. But I got through it.

During those years of living by myself, I never kept foods nearby that might tempt me to binge, such as cereal or ice cream. I did have concerns about living with Kevin as a marriage partner, someone who did not have a problem with food. Kevin kept his kitchen stocked at all times. He loves to cook and to make bread, and cereal is his breakfast of choice. I wondered really just how far advanced I was in my recovery. If we married, I knew he would want to have food in the house. Kevin is naturally lean and can (and does) eat anything he wants. He is also athletic and requires a lot of energy from his food, so he is a big eater. I turned it all over to God. The truth was, if I could not deal with having many different kinds of food in the house, then I was still controlled by my obsession.

Kevin asked me to marry him, I happily accepted, and we set a date for late February. He decided to take an early buyout from his company and relocate to my area, confident he would be able to land a good job in his profession, the rapidly expanding high-tech market. His confidence was confirmed when he received a job offer from a company ten minutes from my business, literally the day before we got married. He started after we returned from our honeymoon.

Kevin owned a beautiful red Chow-Chow dog named Tiger. We had to introduce Tiger and my three cats very carefully! Although they were all to be siblings living under the same roof, we were unsure if they would get along together. Tiger hated cats. The first night Tiger slipped off his leash and spotted Bootsley running through the livingroom of my little house. It turned into a three-ring circus. Cats and fur flew everywhere with Tiger yelping and jumping on the furniture. However, in the days to follow the animals soon began to realize they would have to learn to live with each other in relative peace. Soon they fell into a groove of defiant acceptance, mostly on the cats' part. Tiger would occasionally give chase; at other times, they would simply swat his head as he walked past. All in all, it was quite comical.

Things were going well for us. We found an attractive little fixer-upper close to our jobs and started together down the road of marriage. To my immense relief, storing a lot of food in our house was not a problem. The biggest problem was my misery in working with M. and the total imbalance between my income and hers. I found myself working harder, dealing with so much more and making less than I ever had in my life. I was feeling overwhelmed. Nearly everything that I pulled in went back out for rent, taxes, supplies and the like. Though M. and I had a business agreement it seemed to be working more to her advantage than mine, and she seemed unwilling to change it. I realized that running a business with all its problems is just a part of life—and I can deal with them without running to cereal or ice cream for comfort. I was grateful for that sanity.

M. and I had been in business for over two and one half years by this point. Then, ironically, the biggest blessing happened for Kevin and me. He got laid off from his job. It forced me to ask M. to let me out of the lease. I walked away after months of hard work and an investment of over $30,000 with my loyal clients and one wonderful employee. It was not possible for Kevin and me to exist on the meager earnings I had been taking out of the business. I was free. Now that the business was behind me, I had to address another problem I had been concealing and could no longer ignore—my marriage and relationship with my husband.

CHAPTER 19

TROUBLE ON THE
HOME FRONT

As I said earlier the biggest problem in my marriage was my conflict with M. Once that problem was gone, I realized that Kevin and I had to solve our own communication problems and resolve our different ideas on marriage. In so many ways, Kevin was my "knight in shining armor" and in other ways, my nemesis. Once my dysfunctional business relationship was gone, I still had the challenge of a marital relationship that was creating problems for both of us.

I am extremely independent, and I have never liked having to tell anybody my comings and goings. Well, I was to discover that my husband liked to be informed. Not that he wanted to control what I did, he just liked to know. Also, as an engineer, Kevin was analytical by temperament and could be quite critical. In my opinion, he liked to deal with me as he did an engineering problem. In other words, he would analyze the problem, criticize when necessary, then conclude that the problem should solve itself. In his mind, that would make everything better. He felt that if he challenged every decision I made and pointed out all the potential problems or different ways of doing things, I would then be a better person.

It did not; it made me into an angry person. There was really no ease in our relationship for many years, because he felt that he had to challenge and analyze nearly everything I did. If I bought butter, he asked why I did not buy margarine. When I wanted to replace my $50.00, six-year-old mountain bike that kept losing its chain, he challenged my choice. Are you sure this is the right decision? Do you really need a new bike? It turned into a major discussion. When I wanted to purchase life insurance for $12.60 a month for my own peace of mind, we had one of our biggest arguments. He felt I had acted too impulsively; that I needed to try to get a better deal through a different company rather than just taking the word of the family friend and insurance broker I had been dealing with for seventeen years. I was beginning to get the feeling that my husband had lost faith in my decisions and needed to be in control.

Then we went on the now-famous Mexican vacation. We failed to agree on practically everything. Kevin could not make a decision without comparing and analyzing everything. We had to get the best deal. We went to seven different restaurants one night before he could decide where to eat. By the time he finally decided on one, my patience and tolerance were gone and my anger was out of control. Without knowing it, he would take me to the edge of my tolerance, and than wonder why I would lose my temper and become emotionally upset.

We shopped for new furniture and visited more than twenty different stores before he could make a decision. Fun and spontaneity seemed to have left our marriage. Everything became a chore and a challenge. The more indecisive and analytical he became, the more decisive and short-tempered I became. I felt that we were no longer a team. On that vacation, we finally made a decision to seek marriage counseling.

As soon as we got back, I started making phone calls to find a counselor. True to form, Kevin decided we really did not need counseling; he felt it was too expensive and we could fix whatever problems we had ourselves. I decided to respond with an example to which he could certainly relate: "I may know what the problem is with my car, but that doesn't mean I know how to fix it." Counseling too expensive? "Not as expensive as a divorce," I told him. And I felt that this was where our marriage was heading.

Life is challenging enough. I did not want to come home every night and face insignificant battles in my marriage. I wanted my home to be a haven; I wanted my marriage to be something I enjoyed, and that I could point to with pride. I did not feel that way about it now, and I know Kevin did not either.

We went through several months of counseling. It was a wonderful choice for both of us. We worked through many of our differences, made decisions about how to handle our money, and learned which battles were the really important ones. Obviously the choice between butter or margarine was not one of them—nor was an argument over spending $12.60 a month for insurance. We had to decide which issues were really important to us and worthy of "argument" if there was to be one at all. Most important, we decided that our marriage was far more important to the both of us than any of our individual needs, and that any of those needs would ultimately get met if we put our marriage first. We agreed that the little things would eventually work themselves out. We had to concentrate on the large issues like communication, loyalty, affection; and working and living together as a team.

It took us a couple of years to get through those difficult times in our marriage, but it was definitely worth our efforts.

I know I can totally count on my husband. He has tempered my compulsive nature, and I have taught him the value of being less critical and more generous in his opinions.

Needless to say, for many months I retained a lot of anger and resentment toward M. and the resulting dysfunction of our business. It has been said that Nature will exact a vengeance on those who abuse her, and this may be the case with people. True to M.'s compulsion for spending money she did not have, she ran her once-thriving business into the ground. Two years later she had a tax lien for over $25,000 on the business, and I heard rumors that she owed over $70,000 to suppliers and vendors. She did receive a form of assistance, but at a heavy price. A wealthy woman bailed her out of debt in exchange for major ownership of M.'s still popular, but now financially unhealthy, business. I felt vindicated and, I must confess, a certain measure of elation at hearing about her hardship. On the other hand, these feelings were mixed with a sense of compassion, because it must have been hard for her to relinquish such a major part of a business to which she was so attached.

By this time I had started another business one block from M.'s, and I was enjoying being a sole proprietor. My husband landed a great new job, and I spent the next year getting emotionally and financially on my feet. I took money out of my life insurance policy to renovate an old Victorian house, where I installed a full-service day spa and salon. This put me in direct competition with M., who was only a block away. I had eleven wonderful people working for me. Today, I still have the one employee, Tracy, who worked for me when I was in business with M. It feels good to have someone you can trust and who will be loyal to you for so many years.

Such a relationship has served us both well. Tracy has been with me for over nine years and is such a valuable asset in giving me excellent insight into the selections of new employees. She has watched me open a second location, and has built a great clientele of her own. I have also found another good friend in Radine, who was most helpful in getting my business started. She was always there when I needed her.

I owe my sister, Marilyn, much gratitude in getting my second business started through developing an important liaison between my spa business and the plastic surgeon for whom she works. Through this blending of his profession and our businesses, we were able to create a state-of-the-art spa with advanced medical skin care. I am surrounded by a great staff of women and I am very grateful for that. We are always supportive of each other and enjoy our mutual successes. It is immensely beneficial to work in such a positive environment. And I know it is good for my soul.

Food has now found a proper place in my life. My last binge was over nine years ago. I attribute this to nothing less than putting God first in my life. When I make God my priority, everything falls into place. I eat when I am hungry and enjoy what I am eating. I eat anything I want, and I do not restrict what I eat. However, I do make good choices, and I listen to my body. (I must confess I am still a bit of a sugar fiend, but I try to keep that within reasonable bounds.)

I am grateful every day for the miracle of my restored sanity around food; it truly is a gift of God. I still exercise every day. I walk my dog. I am still an avid biker, and we own all the necessary workout equipment we need at home to use during the winter months. Exercise is as important to me as it has always been; I just do not abuse it any more. I build it into my day, as I do my showering, meditating and other daily routines. Many of our vacations are built around athletic activity. When we went to Ireland a while back, we saw the country on bikes, averaging some 50 miles a day. Both of us still scuba dive and hike. We enjoy being fit and athletic. Life would be pretty empty for me if I could not hike up a mountain in the summer or ski down one in the winter.

Since food is no longer my obsession, I can now put my attention toward far more productive (and definitely not abusive) matters. I can now enjoy my marriage, my perfect niece and nephew, my two businesses, and my new, energetic life. It is amazing how much life unfolds and what good can come into it when you put away your addictions. I know I am never going to be a size three again, and I do not want to be. I am a size eight and have been for over six years now. The main point is that my life is now in balance. Of course, my family tells me I work too much, and I do, but I truly enjoy my work. And I know that I could never have achieved the owning of two healthy businesses if I were still a slave to out-of-control eating.

Life really does open up wonderful opportunities when you allow for them. Once in a while, I catch myself watching someone with an eating disorder, unable to talk about anything but food. I find myself experiencing a whole range of emotions—anger, irritation, and compassion—as I view their obsession. I want to take these people and shake them and make them see that there is so much more to life than the fleeting pleasure (usually followed by pain) of food. And, of course, we are talking about too *much* food. But they must travel their own journey, as I had to travel mine.

I count myself lucky to be married to Kevin, because he is a sensible eater and naturally lean and athletic. I'm afraid the stereotypical couch potato with a can of beer in hand would not be my fancy. Kevin has a stable, solid, cautious personality, which is good for me. His personality complements mine. I would not have lived with a mentally healthy husband if I were addicted. Like does attract like, and once I had reached balance and contentment in my life through spiritual guidance and inner strength, I was guided to someone who was balanced and strong in his own life.

When I look at the good in my life, I feel inclined to pat myself on the back for creating my life as it is today. I truly know that with the help and guidance of God, I am the master of my universe. I feel that the more positive and grateful I am each day, the better the next day will be. Over the past few years I have had a lot of curve balls thrown at me; but now I am able to handle them effectively and still feel at peace with myself.

I believe that a significant part of any recovery program is being of service to those who still suffer. I mention this because I have recently returned to Overeaters Anonymous to serve as best I can those who are suffering as I did. I wrote earlier that when I was involved in OA I found a low success rate for one primary reason: those who received help did not return to help those that needed it. I number myself among them. This flies in the face of the high goals of the OA program. At the time of this writing, I find myself facing new challenges in my life and realize now more than ever that service to others is another important way to serve your own inner growth and happiness.

I have also watched people involved in a twelve-step recovery program who become equally addicted to the meetings. I am all for "whatever it takes" to get a grip on an addiction and move forward. But I know people who have been attending these programs four and five times a week for years and are unable to release themselves even after they have conquered their addiction. They are often prevented from taking a vacation or doing something spontaneously for fear of missing a meeting. To me that isn't recovery, but another form of addiction. If someone is that dependent on a meeting to stay sober or clean after seven or eight years in the program, he or she has not grown much and has really failed to rely on their higher power. Is this not the whole point of recovery? Anyone who has successfully moved past an addiction and truly met themselves on the other, healthier side of their being can relate to my passion.

Life is too beautiful to waste it on an addiction. It does not matter whether that addiction is alcohol, drugs, sex, relationships, food or money. As we move away from our addictions and bring our life into balance, peace of mind begins to grow within us. The greater your peace of mind, the more possibilities will open up in your world. From my own experience I know that when I am the most relaxed and peaceful is when I receive the most inspiration for personal growth, not only for my business but in so many other areas of my life.

At the time of this writing, Kevin and I have been married for slightly over nine years. We have both grown incredibly—both personally and professionally. We have had to put Tiger and Bootsley to sleep. Both of them had inoperable cancers. Our animals are our children and it is always painful to lose one. I still have Theo (my first-born) and Gray, the cat that adopted me. Both Theo and I have been through a lot together—from the time I left the Rader Institute (and 218 pounds), through many jobs and then my road to recovery and weight loss. We adopted another Chow-Chow from a shelter. He keeps me walking, and walking keeps him happy. Marilyn met a wonderful man, and their wedding was a few months after ours.

My mother has never remarried. When asked why, she always says, "Your father is a hard act to follow." I would have to agree. I cannot imagine loving or liking any man as much as I did my father. My younger brother married a woman I adore and they blessed our family with two children. I believe myself to be a wonderful aunt, perhaps better than the mother I never was. My older brother lives in a different city and manages to keep in touch. He recently surprised us all by showing up unannounced to visit each member of the family. That was a gift which pleased us all. I have many blessings. I am grateful every day for my new-found respect for a sensible approach to eating. Food no longer controls my life; I control it.

I have said many times that I would not trade my present peace of mind for a billion dollars if it meant returning to the state I lived in thirteen years ago. I am truly grateful that I found my higher power, God, from which I have been granted the gift of the sanity and peace I longed for so many years ago.

CHAPTER 20

A PROGRAM FOR RECOVERY

Recovery from any controlling addiction is never easy. I suppose if it were, there would be a rapidly diminishing number of addicted people! Unfortunately, that is not the case. In order for us to grow out of an addiction, we must first of all learn to grow inwardly. And by that I mean we must learn to develop some type of spiritual discipline. Living a spiritual life requires that we first have an underlying healthy respect for our physical and mental well-being. Our body and mind have been gifted to us, and it should be our first responsibility to treat them with the reverence they deserve. The ancient adage *mens sana in copore sano* (a sound mind in a sound body) has withstood the test of time with good reason.

The basis for our physical and emotional well-being is spiritual. This may be as simple as saying "no" to someone when it would be far easier (and perhaps temporarily more gratifying) to say "yes." Spirituality means holding your ground, when it might be easier to simply accommodate someone to keep the peace. This does not mean that we must always have our own way; rather, once we know what our real way is—the way we must travel to true health of body and mind—then we must get on that path and stay there. God will take care of the rest.

I know that many of the reasons that I ate excessively were out of a deep well of frustration and an immature wanting to please people. I now realize that the person one must first please is oneself. That is the one to whom we owe our first responsibility. This is not selfishness. It is learning to integrate all of the wonderful parts of our being so that we are complete individuals, not fragmented and isolated beings. Be the best of which you are capable (and you are far more capable than you can possibly imagine!), and life will evolve for you in manifold and wonderful ways.

Inner growth is a continuing process. And the first step is to love and respect who we are. Once we are able to do this, we will never want to mistreat ourselves by overeating, laziness or surrendering to abusive and toxic relationships. There is nothing quite so harmful to our inner spirit as living a life that denies its potential by surrendering to any of these negative influences. If we submit to any of them, we not only insult our spiritual self, but curtail the potential for real inner growth.

In truth, we are all on a journey that requires us to recognize and honor not only ourselves but others who travel with us and assist us in our growth. Of course, there are those who may be harmful to us and betray our trust (and this has happened to me, as you have read in preceding chapters); however, such events should never create so much anger or irritability in us that we take it out on food! If such negative situations present themselves to me, this is when I turn to God and prayer with greater intensity. It is amazing what miracles happen when you surrender to your inner Divinity and seek its help and guidance. "Do unto others as you would have them do unto you" is the rule I sincerely try to follow.

Sometimes I find this rule sorely tested. Only recently I discovered that a senior employee had betrayed my trust by quitting me to work for a competing company after I had spent considerable money to train her. Meanwhile, another senior employee tried to sue me after I had demoted her earlier for improper behavior. All this happened in the middle of a tax audit! Although I experienced a great deal of stress during these events—I am sure my employees were not always too happy with my moods—I was still able to draw upon my inner strengths and not abuse food as I am certain I would have done in earlier years. I know now that if I were still living with an eating disorder I would have never been capable of building the kind of businesses I have or facing the challenges that come with them.

Following are some of the disciplines that have helped me most in overcoming my food addiction:

1. WALKING

This is a great way to start your day. Not only are you able to get your heart going but it is a marvelous way to be alone with your thoughts and ideas for the new day. Not only is it good for the mind, but the spirit as well. And, of course, it is great exercise. I usually walk three miles every morning at a fairly brisk pace. I never miss a day. One added bonus: you meet some wonderful neighbors!

2. Meditation

For me meditation is praying, and praying is thanking God for all the infinite gifts in my life. A grateful heart is a happy heart. I try to meditate every day for an hour. When the weather is good, I sit outside and listen to various meditation CDs from Roger Teel, minister of the Mile Hi Church of Religious Science, or from the Holosync Solution (information on this helpful technique can be found at www.centerpoint .com) or a combination of both. I also found it beneficial to create a little meditation area in my home. I often just sit in my "meditation spot" and in silence wait for guidance and direction from God to select the right path for me to follow.

3. Quigong (Chee-gong)

Quigong is an ancient Chinese energy practice of simple movements to help rejuvenate your internal energy systems. It is a self-healing discipline that seeks to get at the root cause of a problem, not just its symptoms. This technique is known as "The Dragon's Way" and is taught at many yoga and other centers. I have been practicing this for more than a year now and found it to be quite beneficial to my overall health. It also includes ways to eat healthily through consuming healing foods. It has helped me immensely.

4. Eating Well

Make good food choices. Just as you would not put contaminated fuel in your car to cause it to run poorly, why should you put bad fuel in your body? Fruits, vegetables, nuts, and whole grains are some of the best "fuels" for a healthy body. Most foods are fine if you eat them in moderation. Above all, *enjoy* your food and be grateful for it. If you feel guilty about food, is this really being good to yourself? I try to stay faithful to the Quigong way of eating. This involves eating lots of steamed or stir-fried vegetables, nuts, whole grains in moderation, fresh fruits, and lots of watermelon when in season. I seldom pay attention to cook books or diet regimens. Most of them stay too *focused* on food, per se. Isn't that what we are trying to avoid?

At times I feel as if making peace with food was just the first step in this incredible journey of mine. However, I would not trade the challenging events that have unfolded in my life for anything if it meant going back to where I was when I was in the grip of my addiction. As Mary Black, a great singer and songwriter, once said, "Peace of mind is worth any chore."

The peace of mind gained through knowing I can rely on my higher power to guide me is worth all the efforts I have made on my path. I pray that the inner peace I now have may come to any of you who might be struggling with an addiction that is making your life unmanageable. Embark on the journey.

It is worth it!

SOME BOOKS
THAT HAVE HELPED ME

Food for Thought, a part of the Hazelden Meditation Series, Hazelden Foundation, Harper/Hazelden, 1980.

For Today, published by Overeaters Anonymous, Inc., Torrance, CA. This daily guide helped me immensely to get through the really tough times. I highly recommend it.

You Can Heal Your Life, Louise L. Hay, published by Hay House, P.O. Box 5100, Carlsbad, CA. 1984, 1987. A wonderful book for any person in pain and seeking to improve their life. It gave me much help when I needed it most, and particularly when I was just out of treatment.

Love Your Body, Louise L. Hay, 1998. This excellent book contains thirty days of affirmations to guide you toward a healthy, beautiful body. A very helpful addition to any library.

Seven Spiritual Laws of Success, Deepak Chopra, published by Amber Allen Publishing Co., San Rafael, CA. 1994. A book I still love to read often.

Sermon on the Mount, Emmett Fox, published by Harper & Row, 1938. This was one of my father's favorites that helped keep him sober for the remainder of his life.

Science of Mind Textbook, Ernest Holmes, published by Dodd & Mead Co., 1938.

ABOUT THE AUTHOR

BARBARA MCCALMON was inspired to write *Your Weight or Your Life?* by her lifelong struggle with an eating disorder and severe weight problems that began in her preteen years. Even at her thinnest, she was not free from the power that food held over her. The author's time spent in the Rader Institute for Eating Disorders and her ensuing road to recovery gave her the determination to "win" over the disease that controlled her life for so long.

Inspired by this philosophy, McCalmon founded and operated two immensely successful day spas in the Denver area which she has recently decided to sell, allowing her to focus her attention on public speaking and lecturing to those who still suffer from the obsessive power that food has over their lives.

A Colorado native, Barbara and her husband, Kevin, along with their dog Ollie, have built their lives in this beautiful state. Both thrive in the active lifestyle that Colorado provides. This includes hiking, biking, and skiing in the surrounding area.

Barbara is dedicated to her family and practicing the principals she has learned from the Mile Hi Church. She is presently at work completing her first novel, *Blue Eyed Boy*.

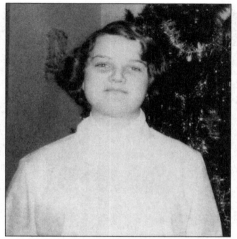

At age thirteen, round and loving food.

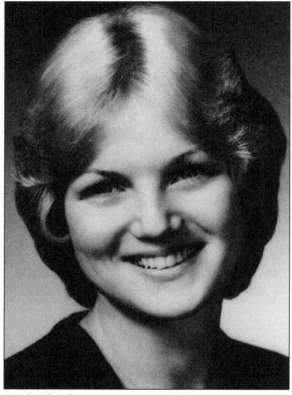

High school senior portrait with an average weight
of 140 pounds during the active years.

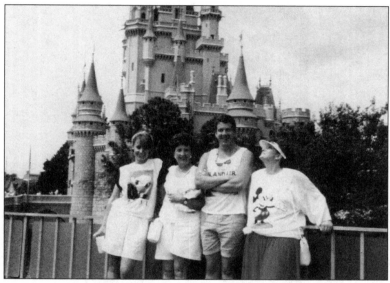

At Disney World with (left to right) my sister, Mom, younger brother, and me, eight months out of the institute, and still very heavy but making progress in mind and body.

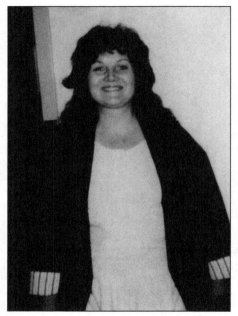

By age twenty-nine, 218 pounds.

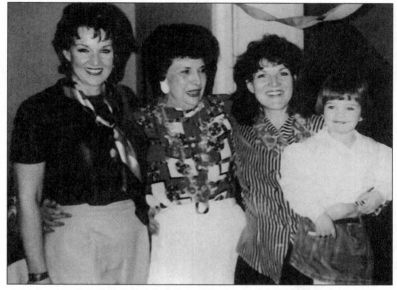

A great day. My fortieth-birthday surprise party with Marilyn, Mom, and my wonderful niece, Cassidy.

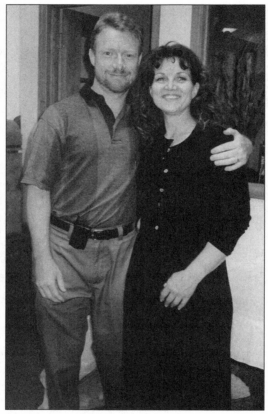

At the grand opening of the Tapestry Spa in
Louisville, Colorado, with my husband, Kevin.